Poultry Inspection

2nd Edition

Anatomy, physiology and disease conditions

A Grist

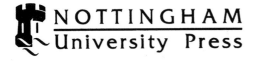

NOTTINGHAM
University Press

Nottingham University Press
Manor Farm, Main Street, Thrumpton
Nottingham NG11 0AX, United Kingdom
www.nup.com

NOTTINGHAM

First published 2006
© A Grist

British Library Cataloguing in Publication Data
Poultry Inspection - 2nd Edition
Anatomy, physiology and disease conditions
A Grist

ISBN-10:   1-904761-53-4
ISBN-13:   978-1-904761-53-2

Disclaimer

Typeset by Nottingham University Press, Nottingham
Printed and bound by Hobbs the Printers, Hampshire, England

INTRODUCTION

This book is designed to provide notes for students undertaking the Royal Society for the Promotion of Health (RSPH) examination in Poultry Meat Inspection, and as a revision guide for students undertaking other courses in which knowledge of poultry anatomy, diseases and conditions is required such as Veterinary Courses, Environmental Health and Poultry Science.

It is hoped that this may also provide source material for the theoretical training of abattoir staff to undertake post-mortem inspection of poultry in licensed premises under the supervision of the Official Veterinarian as is currently allowed under European law.

Following the success of the first edition of Poultry Inspection, this second edition, updated and augmented was produced. Poultry Inspection was the first book I wrote in the series published by Nottingham University Press and as such I was unsure what others would require of it, or indeed how much information I should give. Since its publication in 2004 I feel that I have a better idea of what I, and others, expect of the book. To that end I have replaced a large number of the diagrams with labelled photographs and expanded the Anatomy section to give what I hope will be a clearer and better understanding of the subject. The general layout of the book has been further altered to follow the other books in the series including Bovine Meat Inspection and Ovine Meat Inspection due to the positive feedback received.

The Diseases of Poultry section has been updated and now includes photographs of some of the conditions and begins with a basic explanation of the disease process and the body's response. The diseases and conditions are listed in alphabetical order rather than in any order of incidence or priority as these factors can be subject to annual and seasonal variation. The parasites section has been improved by the addition of photographs, most of these kindly supplied by Daniel Parker BVMS Cert PMP MRCVS of the Slate Hall Veterinary Practice, Cambridge.

Having tutored on the subject of poultry inspection and been asked to explain to various students a method for performing post mortems on suspect birds, this has been included as a separate section with explanation and photographs. This section is only intended for guidance, as each person finds their own methods of examination which they are comfortable performing.

I hope that I have recorded all the professionals that provided advice and encouragement in the acknowledgments section, and sincerely hope that this edition fulfils expectations.

AUTHOR DISCLAIMER

I must add that the judgments are my own views. They are based on experience of Poultry Inspection, both broiler and organic/free range systems, and through consultation with others.

A Grist

ACKNOWLEDGEMENTS

This second edition would not have been possible without the support and encouragement of the following people; especially Rita Hinton and Dr Leisha Hewitt of the Continuing Education Department at Langford School of Veterinary Science. Malcolm Morris BVSc MRCVS, retired Principal Veterinary Surgeon of the Meat Hygiene Service for assistance above and beyond the call of duty, and for teaching the meat inspection students at Langford that they could and should make a difference. Dr Sophia Rizvi MRCVS of DEFRA for advice, friendship and comments.

Thanks are also due to Daniel Parker BCVMS Cert PMP MRCVS of the Slatehall Veterinary Practice, Cambridge for his professionalism, allowing the use of his photographs and providing advice and encouragement whenever it was required.

Martin Evans, Area Manager and Gavin Morris MRCVS Regional Veterinary Adviser, both of the Meat Hygiene Service, and Peter Costema of the Association of Meat Inspectors for all their support. I would also like to thank Mike Edwards DVMS MRCVS, the lead Official Veterinarian at the plant at which I am currently based, and Gordon Gait, Senior Meat Inspector, for their patience during the researching of this book.

Special mention must be made of John Steer, Jane Jones, Louise Cotter, Carol Loud, Doris Jones, Andy Jones, Margaret Butterfield, Jason Chivers, Terry Woolland, Sue Coombs, Matt Kosma, June Westall, Robin James, Edward Staples, Sylvia Ryall, Sue Robertson, Sophia D'Costa, Ismatullah Baluj and Susan Hopkins without whom I would not have been able to produce my own photographs for this book. Mr Tony Hack for dealing with constant requests for the more unusual photographs and for driving across country to deliver them and the occasional carcase I would be interested in. Mr Andrew Oatley of Paxcroft Farm for providing birds for the photographs of the female reproductive system.

Again, Sarah Keeling, Sarah Mellor and Ros Webb of Nottingham University Press have been paragons of tolerance, patience, support and encouragement.

My children George, Elizabeth and Henry, who provided encouragement and edited photographs, helped prepare samples including the skeleton, and provided a level of enthusiasm for the books and subject matter that kept me going. The pride they have shown in the books produced to date is a mirror of the pride I have in them.

Most thanks as always goes to my wife, Grace, who kept an environment where writing books was possible, proof read each book I have written, poured through over 4000 photographs for this book alone, became a sounding board for ideas, provided advice when asked and still remains supportive despite the time taken up in authoring this series.

DEDICATION

I have always held the opinion, during my time as a Meat Hygiene Inspector, abattoir manager and lecturer that the food that I inspect should be fit for my own children to eat. If you would not feed it to your own children, you should not expect the consumer to feed it to theirs.

To that end I dedicate this to my wife Grace and my children George, Elizabeth, Henry and Harriette.

In fond memory of Dr Des Cole
Thank you for the opportunity to write

CONTENTS

DIAGRAM LIST

PHOTOGRAPH LIST

Section One
Anatomy and Physiology

Section Two
Diseases of Poultry

Section Eight
Processing Conditions

[1] Authors Own Photograph Library
[2] Courtesy of D.Parker BVMS Cert PMP MRCVS
     Slate Hall Veterinary Practice, Cambridge
[3] Courtesy of M. Morris BVSc MRCVS
[4] Courtesy of Mr Tony Hack
[5] Courtesy of G. Hayes BVMS Cert PMP MRCVS
     Slate Hall Veterinary Practice, Cambridge

FOREWORD TO FIRST EDITION

Poultry meat is now the major meat eaten in the UK, but for many years the post-mortem inspection of poultry was considered of secondary importance to the post-mortem inspection of the red meat species. However, the sheer scale and volume of the poultry meat industry now demands that the post-mortem inspection is carried out with an efficiency that is compatible with the throughput of the industry.

To affect this, the staff undertaking the post-mortem inspection must be trained to a high degree and have knowledge of an increasing number of diseases and conditions encountered in the intensification of the poultry industry. This book will provide an easy reference guide for the student and qualified inspector alike.

What Andy Grist has done is collate all the information accumulated during his experience as a student, inspector and teacher and reproduce it in book form. What pleases me is that he has added information which gives the reader an appetite to read on and in doing so increases our understanding of the subject.

Many of the conditions seen at post-mortem inspection of poultry are due in part to the unique anatomy and physiology of avian species and this has been explained very well.

I have no doubt that this book will be essential reading for our students of the future and its success will be just reward for the hard work that has resulted in its production.

Malcolm Morris BVSc MRCVS
14 September 2003

ANATOMY/
PHYSIOLOGY

1

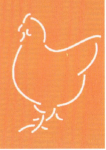

EXTERNAL ANATOMY

The modern fowl is a result of selective breeding over hundreds of years. Broiler chickens are designed to grow as fast as possible, they eat to capacity, not to need, and reach slaughter age at about 37-40 days. The internal and external anatomy has obviously evolved for flight, they have a short, rigid body with a centralized centre of gravity, relatively light heads, flexible necks and their forelimbs have been modified to become wings.

In terms of colour, broilers have white feathers and layer hens have brown, the latter having been based on the Rhode Island Red.

THE HEAD

In the mature bird, the sexual characteristics are pronounced, these being a fleshy **comb** across the top of the head, **wattles** from the base of the beak and prominent **earlobes**. These characteristics are more marked in males than in females. Broiler chickens are immature, but will possess the rudimentary features of the adult.

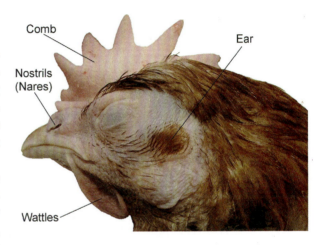

External features of the head

The eyes are large in comparison with mammals, in the live bird the size is obscured by the upper and lower eyelids. A third eyelid, the nictitating membrane, moves across the eye from front to back during blinking, sweeping horizontally across the eye. The loss of the nictitating blink reflex is commonly used as an indication of the successful application of an electroplectic stun.

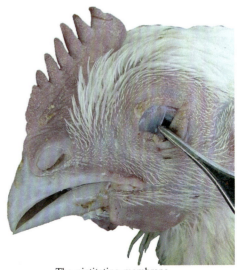

The nictitating membrane

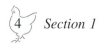

The ear has no external auricle to collect sound. The beak is pliable in the immature bird, but becomes increasingly harder with maturity, and is formed from keratin, a substance similar to the fingernails of humans.

FEATHERS

These are thought to have originally been scales modified to regulate the body temperature that underwent further alteration to enable flight. The feathers grow from follicles in the skin, similar to mammalian hair growth; these large crypts can be colonized by

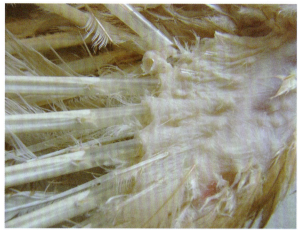

pathogens. The mature feather consists of a hollow quill (**calamus**) that continues into a shaft (**rachis**) from which barbs branch off with interlocking barbules forming the feather vane.

There are four types of feather found on birds:

Down Feathers – are found close to the skin and have no barbules.

Filoplumes – Have long shafts with little vane and are used for display.

Flight Feathers – These have a long rachis and are attached to the major limb bones. Primary and secondary flight feathers (**remiges**) are found on the wings and the remiges used for steering are found on the tail.

Contour feathers – These form the shape and aerodynamics of the bird. They lack interlocking barbules and also act as insulation.

A contour feather, with a second 'afterfeather' thought to increase insulation.

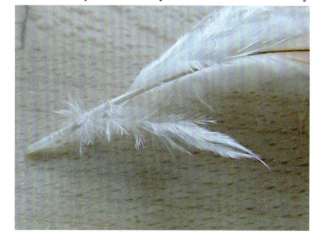

The skin is not completely covered in contour feathers; the feather follicles are arranged in tracts over the skin known as **pterylae,** the spaces in between, usually covered with down feathers and semiplumes, are known as **apteria**.

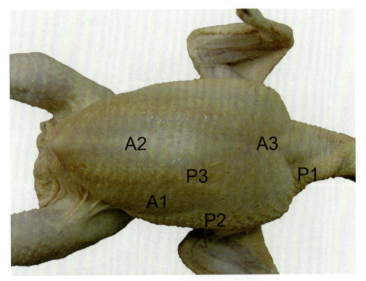

A few of the Pterylae and Apteria of a plucked carcase.
Pterylae - P1:Cervical.P2: Pectoral. P3: Sternal
Apteria – A1: Pectoral. A2: Sternal. A3: Ventral cervical

SKIN

The skin is loosely attached and has a poor blood supply when compared to mammals. There are no sweat glands in poultry. The outer skin, or epidermis, is composed of two layers or strata; the surface strata, (the *stratum corneum)* and the lower strata, (the *stratum germinativum*), the latter of which is made up of three further layers. Dead skin cells are shed continuously and are replaced by the next layer. Skin cells germinate from the lower, basal layer of the *stratum germinativum* and mature as they move through the intermediate and transitional layers to the *stratum corneum.*

PREEN GLAND

At the base of the tail is situated the preen or **uropygial gland**. This is a bi-lobed sebaceous gland, producing sebum, an oily secretion composed of fat and skin cells. This is secreted from two openings at the top of a cone of skin and is carried to the rest of the body by the beak. This substance is used to maintain the condition of the feathers and to provide waterproofing in aquatic species such as ducks.

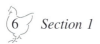

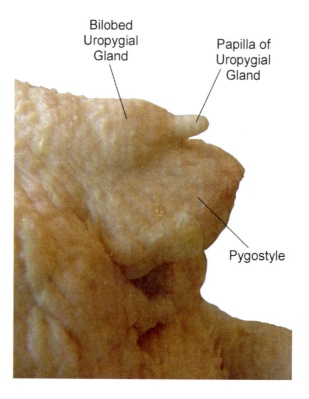

Bilobed
Uropygial
Gland

Papilla of
Uropygial
Gland

Pygostyle

Lateral view of pygostyle and uropygial gland

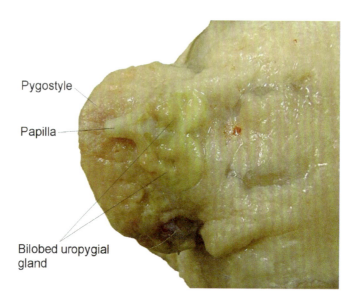

Pygostyle

Papilla

Bilobed uropygial
gland

Dorsal view – skin reflected

SKELETAL STRUCTURE

The bones of the fowl are comparatively light and strong, the skeleton of birds comprises the axial skeleton (head, vertebrae, ribs and sternum) and the peripheral or appendicular skeleton (the limb bones.)

THE STRUCTURE OF BONES

Bone is a collagen matrix containing mineral salts, chiefly calcium phosphate, and various cells including osteoclasts and osteoblasts. The deposition of mineral salts within the matrix is controlled by osteoblasts. Mineral reabsorbtion and release of the minerals into the blood is attributed to the large, mononucleated osteoclasts. These cells work in balance, their activity being controlled by parathyroid hormone (PTH) secreted by the parathyroid gland in response to fluctuation in the serum- calcium level of the blood. If this level decreases more hormone is released having the effect of increasing the activity of the osteoclasts whilst decreasing the osteoblast activity and hence subsequently increasing the calcium in the blood. This deposition and reabsorbtion of mineral salts of the bone is a continual process. Bones have a connective tissue membranous covering, the periosteum, which has bone-forming properties and, through fusion with muscular connective tissue, anchors the muscle to the bone. Under the periosteum is the dense, or compact bone, which in the long bones forms a hollow shaft containing marrow and spongy bone. Marrow occurs in two forms, red and yellow, and is a combination of blood vessels and connective tissue containing fat and blood producing cells. Red marrow produces blood cells such as erythrocytes and leukocytes; yellow marrow is formed mainly from fatty tissue. Spongy or cancellous bone is usually found at the extremities of long bones and is composed of thin intersecting layers of bone. The articular cartilage has a bluish white colour and is also known as hyaline cartilage due to its glassy appearance. The epiphyseal cartilage represents the site at which bone growth increases the length of the long bones. The avian long bones usually contain diverticula of the respiratory system making them light, and only possess a thin cortex of compact bone leading to the necessity for a 'scaffold like' mesh of bone known as trabeculae to increase the strength of the bones.

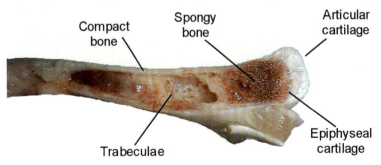

Section through a broiler humerus

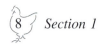

THE AXIAL SKELETON

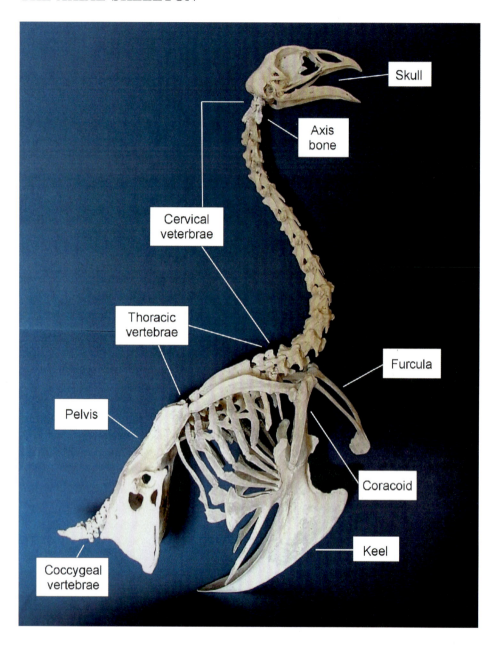

The skull is light, the upper and lower jaw (mandible) contain no teeth, allowing the lower mandible to be incredibly light compared to mammals as it does not have to withstand the forces exerted in the process of biting and chewing. The eye socket is large.

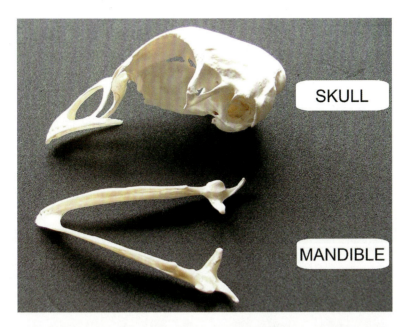

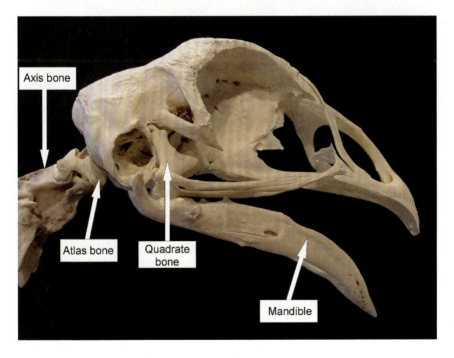

The skull, atlas and axis bone of an adult male broiler. The quadrate bone forms part of the complex hinge of the mandible that allows flexation of the upper jaw.

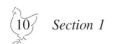

The spine, or vertebral column is composed of bones called vertebrae that are grouped into regions. Some vertebrae are fused together, providing strength and rigidity, the others move in relation to their neighbour (articulate). There are 13/14 **cervical vertebrae** as opposed to the 7 found in the neck of mammals. This forms the basis of an extremely flexible neck. The first cervical vertebra is called the axis bone about which the skull rotates, allowing high mobility of the skull in contrast to that of mammals. The last two cervical vertebrae articulate with the first two ribs.

The four **thoracic vertebrae** form the rear wall of the chest cavity (thorax). The first three vertebrae are fused together with the last cervical vertebrae and are immobile forming the notarium, the fourth thoracic vertebrae is mobile.

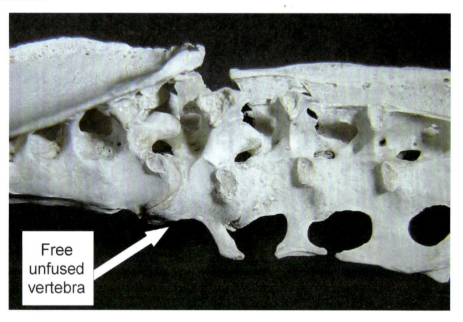

Free unfused vertebra

The four **lumbar vertebrae**, five **sacral vertebrae** and six **caudal vertebrae** are all fused together to form a structure called the **synsacrum**. The **ilium, ischium and pubis** bones are fused together with the synsacrum to form the **pelvis**.

The six **coccygeal vertebrae** are small, except the last, the **pygostyle** that is flattened and forms the tailbone.

There are seven pairs of **ribs**; two joined to the last two cervical vertebrae, four to the thoracic and one pair to the first lumbar vertebrae. The first two ribs articulating with the cervical vertebrae do not reach the sternum. The remaining ribs comprise two sections, the vertebral and sternal segments. With the exception of the first and seventh ribs, the vertebral segment has a small, flat outgrowth called the uncinate process over the adjacent rib.

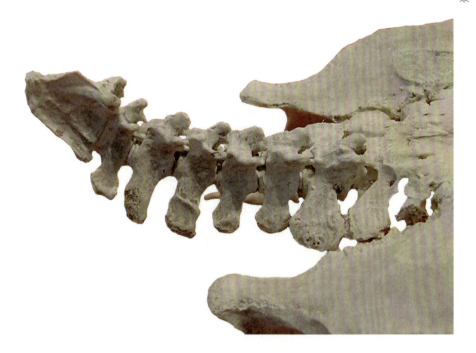

Coccygeal vertebrae, terminating at the flattened pygostyle

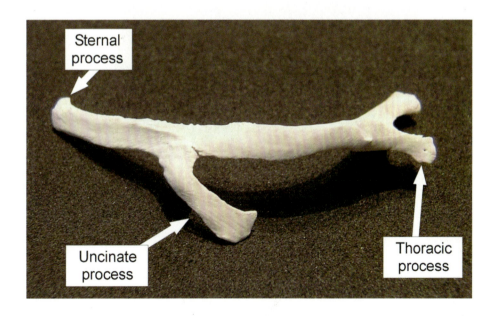

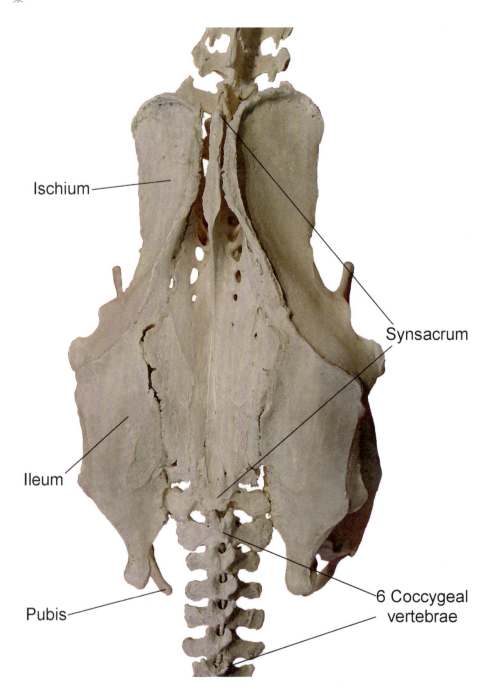

Ischium

Synsacrum

Ileum

Pubis

6 Coccygeal vertebrae

The Avian Pelvis and Synsacrum

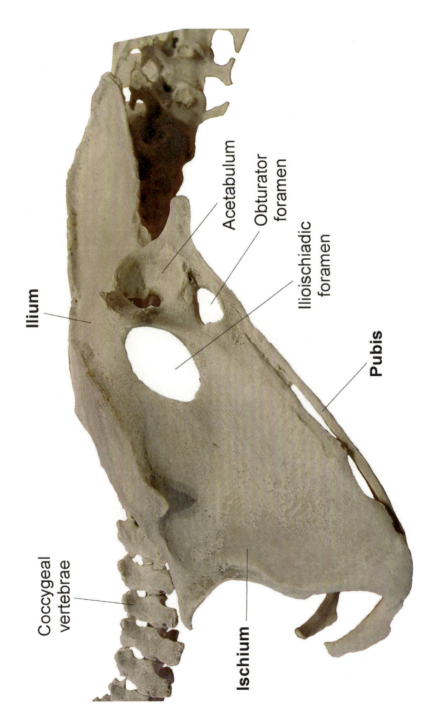

Avian pelvis – lateral view

The **sternum** is keel shaped allowing for the attachment of the large pectoral muscle groups and articulates cranially with the coracoid and with the sternal segments of the ribs via the costal facets.

The pectoral girdle is made up of two **clavicles** forming the furcula (wishbone), the two **coracoid** bones, and two **scapula** (shoulder blades). The coracoid bone is absent in mammals, this girdle produces a specialized bracing structure allowing for a wide range of movement including rotation of the humerus. At the point where the three bones join, a canal (Triosseal canal) is formed through which the tendon of the supracoracoideus muscle passes to attach to the periosteum of the humerus producing the upstroke of the wing on contraction.

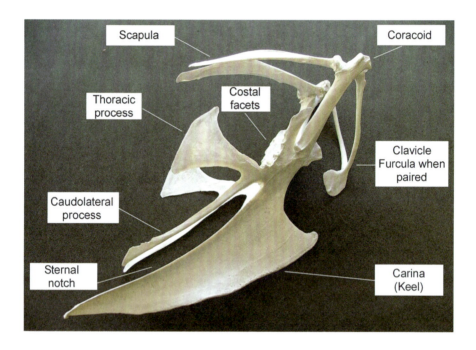

Avian sternum and pectoral girdle

The make up of the axial skeleton is an adaptation to assist in flight, the skeleton is rigid but light with fused vertebrae and interlocking areas, the sternum has a pronounced keel for anchoring the enlarged breast muscles. The head is relatively light, the flexible long neck assists in feeding and balance, and the body is short with a centralized centre of gravity.

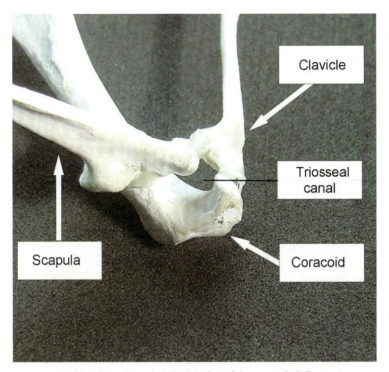

The triosseal canal at the junction of the pectoral girdle

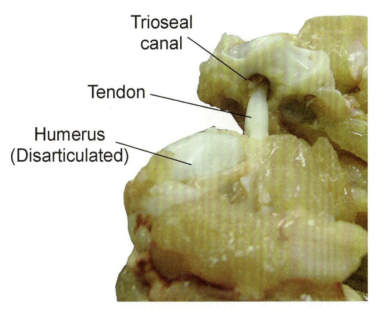

Partially dissected wing – illustrating the tendon of the supracoracoideus muscle

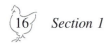

THE APPENDICULAR SKELETON

THE WING

The shoulder blade (**scapula**) is connected at one end to the clavicle/coracoid junction; the remaining length runs along the side of the vertebrae and is joined to the axial skeleton by muscles and ligaments. The **coracoid** bone acts as a strong brace between the shoulder joint and the sternum, providing additional support for the forces exerted during the up and down strokes of the wing. The **humerus** is a pneumatic bone, part of the internal structure incorporating an outgrowth or diverticulum of the intraclavicular air sac, part of the respiratory system. The last few wrist bones (carpals) are fused to the metacarpals, which terminate in three digits.

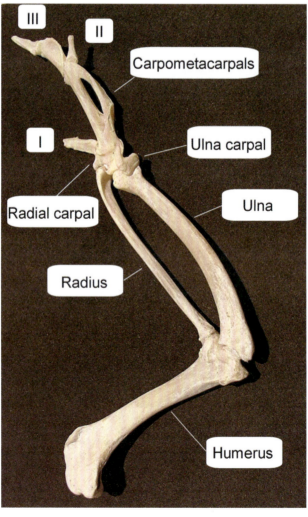

Avian wing

THE HINDLIMB

The **femur** articulates with a cup shaped socket in the pelvis called the **acetabulum**, there is a small kneecap (**patella**) at the other end of this bone. The **tibia** is fused to the ankle bones (tarsus) forming the **tibiotarsus**, the poorly developed **fibula** extends three quarters of the length of the tibiotarsus (drumstick). The remaining ankle bones are fused to form the **metatarsus** from which a rearward projecting spur grows in males.

There are four toes (**digits**) formed by **phalanges**. The first digit projects rearward and comprises 2-3 phalanges. The remaining three digits face forward and comprise 3 phalanges (2nd digit), 4 phalanges (3rd digit) and 5 phalanges (4th digit), the last phalange on each digit forms the basis of the claw.

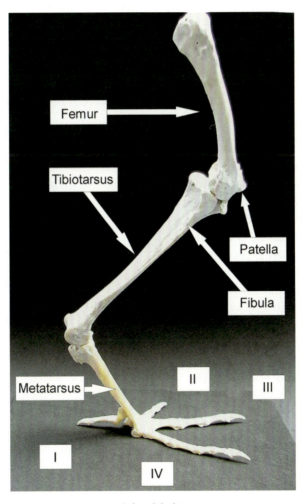

Avian right leg

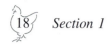

FEET

The feet of poultry possess a single metatarsal pad composed of subcutaneous fatty (adipose) tissue that forms the plantar surface of the foot. Further digital pads are found under the phalanges of each digit. As the plantar surface of the foot is in permanent contact with the ground it has to be considered as a point of pathogen entry should the integrity of the skin be compromised either through injury or contact dermatitis (see pododermatitis).

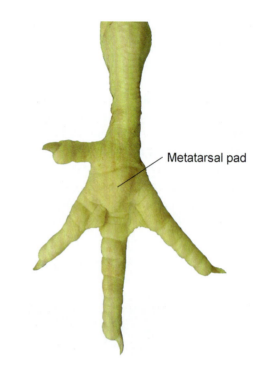

Metatarsal pad

JOINTS

The articulating areas between bones (humerus/radius for example) are examples of synovial joints. The area of the joint is surrounded by a capsule (articular capsule) the inner surface of which consists of a membrane (synovial membrane). The articular capsule contains synovial fluid, a plasma-like fluid secreted by the synovial membrane that lubricates moving parts and nourishes the cartilage.

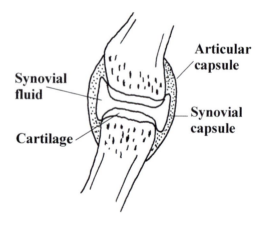

MUSCULATURE

The type and size of the muscles in poultry have evolved specifically to enable and sustain flight, this evolution being enhanced by breeding to increase the proportion of breast muscle to suit consumption.

INTRODUCTION

Muscle is the reason that the meat animals are reared and slaughtered; the post mortem changes that occur in muscle converting it to meat. In the live animal, muscle is found anchored to the skeletal frame providing posture, an ability to move and protection for the internal organs. It is also present internally to provide movement in the viscera and to provide valves to regulate flow, achieving this by converting the chemical energy of ATP (Adenosine triphosphate) to mechanical energy. There are three types of muscle; skeletal muscle, cardiac muscle, and smooth muscle, each possessing different characteristics.

SKELETAL MUSCLE

This is also known as striated muscle and is under semi voluntary control of the nervous system and generally contracts around a fulcrum to facilitate movement about a joint.

ANATOMY OF MUSCLE

Muscle is composed of individual long muscle fibres enclosed by a collagenous membrane, the endomysium, grouped into bundles surrounded by a second membrane called the perimysium. These bundles are further enclosed by the epimysium to form the muscle proper. The epimysium membrane extends past the termination of the muscle fibres to form the tendons that attach the muscles to the bone via the periosteum.

FIBRES

Fibres are formed by the fusion of muscle cells (myoblasts) and hence each fibre contains numerous nuclei and mitochondria. Each fibre contains filaments of protein, the interaction of which in the presence of ATP coverts chemical energy into mechanical energy. Thick filaments are formed by the protein myosin, a protein that contains areas that have an affinity for bonding with ATP and also the protein forming the thinner filaments actin. The term striated muscle is given as, microscopically, bands are visible within the muscle fibre which corresponds to the degree of overlap of these protein filaments in a given area.

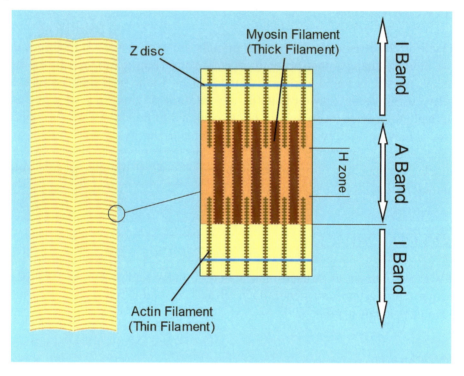

The banding noted in the muscle is given nomenclature, the dark bands are due to the thick filaments of myosin and are termed the A-band, and conversely the I-band is due to the presence of the thinner actin filaments. The area where the two types of filaments do not overlap is called the H-zone. The I-band is bisected by the Z-disc which is a band of non-contractile protein to which the myofibrils are attached; the area between two Z-discs forms the sarcolemma, the functional contractile unit of muscle.

ATP- ADENOSINE TRIPHOSPHATE

ATP is a compound formed by the hydrolysis of nucleic acids known as a nucleotide. It exists in all cells of the body and provides the main energy storage unit, a type of battery that stores energy in the form of high-energy phosphate bonds on the molecule. During muscular contraction the ATP molecule breaks the bond between the actin and myosin filaments but looses a phosphate group in the process releasing energy. The ATP now converts to adenosine diphosphate (ADP). A small amount of ATP is stored in muscle cells; once this has been exhausted the muscle fibre will fatigue as the lactic acid level raises and will cease to function. The replacement of ATP is achieved in three ways, each method producing a phosphate bond to convert ADP to ATP; cellular respiration, conversion of creatine phosphate, and conversion of glycogen. When these methods are exhausted the myosin/actin bonds become permanent.

Cellular respiration is the main method of producing enough ATP to meet the demands of the muscle during prolonged activity and for the conversion of lactic acid to glycogen. Glycogen is stored in muscle fibres, and through the glycolytic pathway reaction, converts ADP to ATP by breakdown of lactic acid. Creatine phosphate reacts with ADP to produce ATP and creatine. These latter reactions are finite; once they have been exhausted cellular respiration provides the energy for ATP production in the muscle.

CONTRACTION

On receiving stimulus from the nerve the myosin head attracts the actin toward it and binds with it, drawing the unfixed thin filament along the fixed thick filament. ATP then breaks this bond and the actin rebinds at the next available myosin head further down the thick filament and the process repeats having the effect of shortening the sarcomere in a gear toothed or ratchet-like manner. During contraction the A-band (the darker band) remains the same size, the I-band shortens as the Z-discs are pulled toward each other.

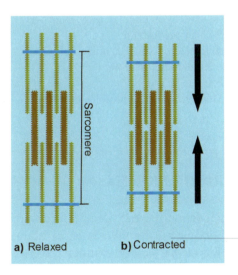

a) Relaxed   b) Contracted

FIBRE TYPES

Two types of fibre are found in a muscle group, Type I (red fibres) and Type II (white fibres) that have different characteristics. The combination of these fibres within a muscle determines that muscles efficiency for the tasks required of it. Red muscle fibres, such as are predominant in the legs of poultry, are smaller than white muscle fibres and contain large amounts of fat,small amounts of glycogen and have a good blood supply. As these fibres use fat as an energy source rather than the carbohydrate used by white muscle fibres, and fat supplies more energy (calories) per unit weight than carbohydrate, red muscle fibres are suited to sustained exertion. In hummingbirds the breast muscles are almost entirely formed of these fibres.

White muscle fibres, such as are predominant in the breast of poultry have a poor blood supply, little fat and high levels of glycogen. These muscles are used for short, powerful contractions and suffer fatigue rapidly. These large breast muscles are attached to the enlarged keel of the sternum and to the humerus and comprise two muscles, the **pectoralis major**, used for the powerful down stroke of the wings, which covers the **supracoracoideus** muscle, which is used for the return upstroke.

The pectoral muscles account for approximately 13-15% of the mass of a broiler chicken.

Type I Fibre	Type II Fibre
Red fibre (Slow Twitch)	White Fibre (Fast Twitch)
Large number of mitochondria	Low number of mitochondria
Dependent on cellular respiration ATP	Dependent on Glycolytic ATP
Rich in myoglobin	Low in myoglobin
Activated by small diameter (slow conducting) neurons	Activated by large diameter (fast conducting) neurons
Fatigue resistant	Used for rapid contraction
More prevalent in muscles of posture	Fatigue easily
	More dominant in muscles used for rapid movement

RIGOR MORTIS

Rigor mortis, the 'death stiffening' that occurs after death is the permanent bonding of the myosin/actin filaments once the available ATP is exhausted due to the lack of cellular respiration. The process of rigor mortis has three phases: A **delay phase** during which time available ATP is used within the muscle fibre to prevent myosin/actin bonding. An **onset phase** during which time the cellular respiration ATP is exhausted and the pool of ATP from creatine phosphate and glycolysis are used up and permanent rigor myosin/actin bonds are formed, and a final **completion phase** where the regeneration of ATP ceases and the myosin/actin filaments become fully bonded. These bonds eventually break due to the lower pH conditions that occur in the carcase. It is worth mentioning that the hardening of fat is not due to rigor but to the lowering of temperature.

NERVE SUPPLY

Each individual muscle fibre is served by an axon that branches from a motor neuron (see nerves types and function in Nervous System section). Stimulation of the motor neuron creates contraction within every fibre served by the branches of its axon, therefore muscles requiring precise control will be served by many neurons with few branches, and large muscles can be controlled by few motor neurons with many branches

SMOOTH MUSCLE

Smooth muscle, also known as visceral muscle is found within the walls of the hollow structures of the body with the notable exception of the heart. This tissue is under involuntary control of the autonomic nervous system.

Contraction of smooth muscle alters the dimension of the structures including the diameter of arteries, the peristaltic motion of the intestines, the diameter of the bronchi, contraction of the urinary bladder during urination, and contraction of the uterus during parturition.

Unlike cardiac and skeletal muscle there are no visible strata within smooth muscle, although it still contains the sliding filaments of actin and myosin but fixed to the cell membrane rather than a Z-disc. Smooth muscle comprises single cells that possess contractile properties. The contraction of smooth muscle is partially involuntary as is cardiac muscle, but can also be stimulated by motor neurons and the presence of hormones. For example the presence of bile in the small intestine has a triggering effect on the peristaltic movement of the intestinal smooth muscle.

CARDIAC MUSCLE

The heart muscle, cardiac muscle, is a specialised form of musculature and is only partly controlled by the autonomic system which has the ability to increase or decrease the rate of contraction but not the act of contraction itself. As with skeletal muscle it appears striated microscopically and contains the sarcomeres associated with skeletal muscle. Cardiac muscle is differentiated from skeletal muscle tissue in unique ways; the two main differences are by-products of the method of function of the heart muscle. Firstly the cardiac muscle is formed by single cells containing a single nucleus as opposed to the multi-nucleated fusion of myoblasts that form skeletal muscle. The second notable difference is that the myofibrils of actin and myosin are branched in cardiac muscle and interlock with those of adjacent fibres to form immensely strong junctions that prevent the fibres separating during the forceful contractions associated with a heart beat.

The contraction of the heart muscle is set up by the fibres themselves, the contraction of one sarcomere initialising contraction of its neighbour via gap junctions, thereby creating a wave effect of contraction starting at the atrium and proceeding down the ventricle forcing blood from the heart. The nervous supply to the heart simply offers only modulation of this beat either speed or strength. The table below illustrates the basic difference between cardiac and skeletal muscle.

Skeletal Muscle	Cardiac Muscle
Multi-nucleated, fusion of myoblasts	Single celled fibres, single nucleus
ATP derived from three sources, creatine phosphate, glycogen, and cellular respiration	ATP almost exclusively via cellular respiration, thus more mitochondria
Myofibrils separated	Myofibrils branched and interlocked
Motor nerve stimulates contraction	Motor nerve modulates contraction
Glycogen stores ten times larger than quantity of ATP stored	Small amount of glycogen stored

MAJOR MUSCLE GROUPS OF POULTRY

There are approximately 170 muscles in chicken, including:

Neck
Longus coli

Wing
Rhomboideus – protracts the wing.
Latissimus dorsi – retracts the wing.
Deltoideus – extends and flexes the shoulder joint.
Triceps- extends trailing edge and flexes elbow joint.
Biceps- Extends leading edge and flexes elbow joint.

Breast
Pectoralis major
Supracoracoideus

Leg
Iliotibialus- major external thigh muscle.
Semitendonosus – back of leg extending to back bone, (preen gland situated above the point of attachment to backbone).

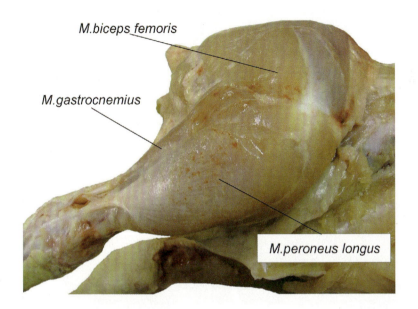

Major muscles of the leg

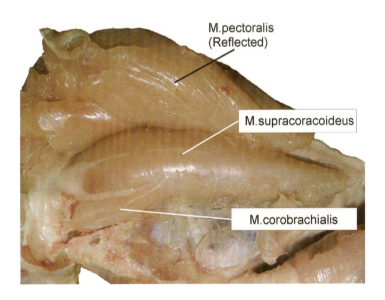

Breast muscles

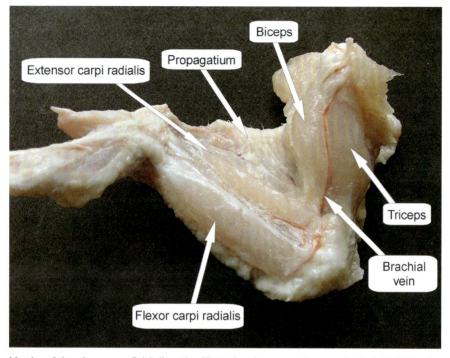

Muscles of the wing – superficial dissection illustrating the propagatium, an elastic fold of skin that increases the surface area of the wing

DIGESTIVE SYSTEM

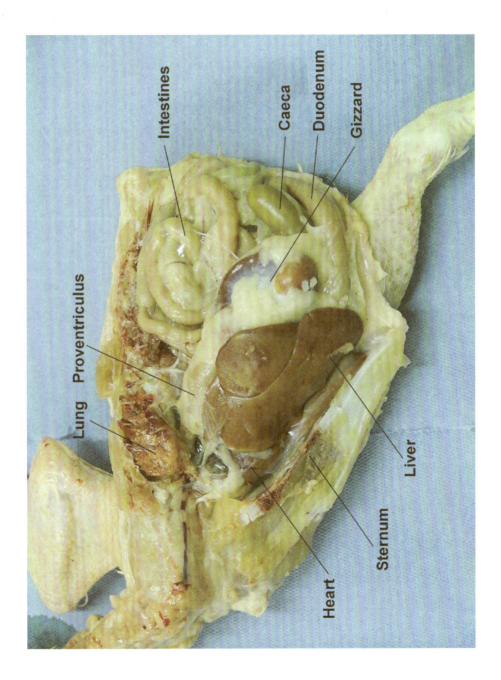

Cross section of a plucked broiler chicken

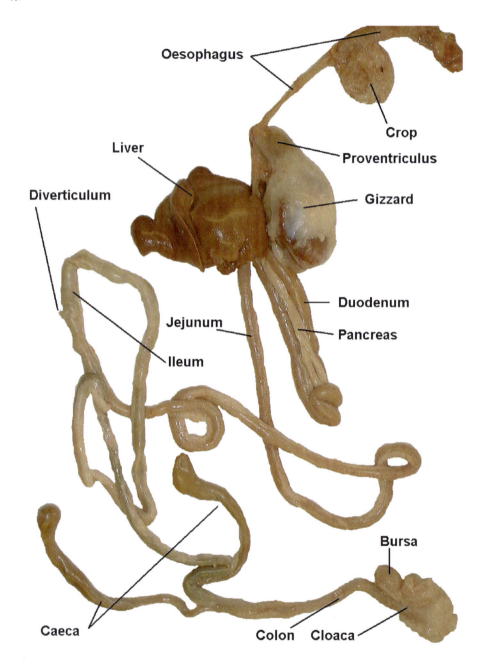

Oesophagus

Crop

Liver

Proventriculus

Diverticulum

Gizzard

Duodenum

Jejunum

Pancreas

Ileum

Bursa

Caeca

Colon Cloaca

Avian Digestive System

The digestive system of poultry is basically a tube, beginning at the mouth and ending at the vent. Food is taken in (ingested), lubricated, mixed with acid and enzymes, ground up and the resultant paste is passed to the small intestines where nutrients and water are absorbed before any waste matter is excreted. **Oesophagus**. Food is taken in via the mouth and mixed with saliva to lubricate it. Birds possess no teeth so the food is swallowed whole as a 'ball' (bolus). The bolus moves down the oesophagus by gravity and a wave-like contraction of the muscles (peristalsis), which are arranged both lengthways and in a circular manner down the oesophagus.

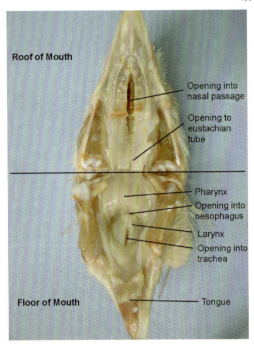

Crop. The bolus then enters the crop where it is stored if the stomach is full. A certain amount of softening and fermentation may occur here. The crop is situated just outside the entrance of the chest cavity (thoracic inlet) and is an expansion of the oesophagus. A further section of the oesophagus connects the crop to the proventriculus within the thoracic cavity.

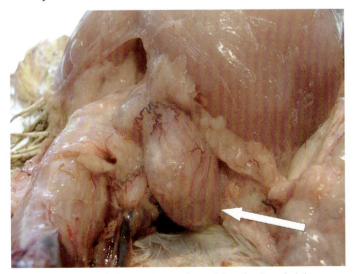

The position of the crop (arrowed) cranial to the thoracic inlet

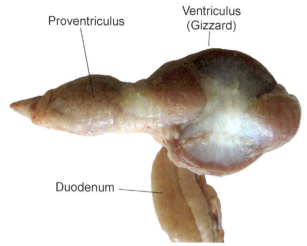

Proventriculus

Ventriculus
(Gizzard)

Duodenum

Proventriculus. The food now enters the proventriculus, the 'true stomach'. The internal surface is lined with cells in the form of columns that produce hydrochloric acid (HCl) and an enzyme (pepsin). This starts the process of breaking down the protein constituent of food into simple components.

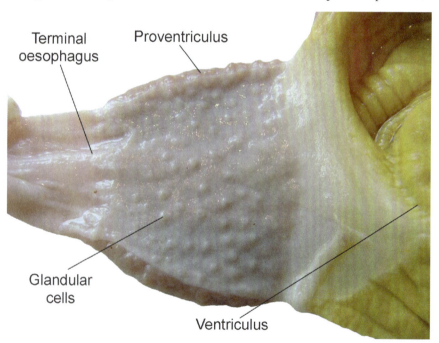

Terminal
oesophagus

Proventriculus

Glandular
cells

Ventriculus

Ventriculus . (**Gizzard**). The food, mixed with these gastric juices passes to the gizzard. The internal surface of the gizzard is covered with a hard, yellowish, ridged lining called the *cutica gastrica* secreted by cells within the gizzard lining. The muscles of the gizzard are arranged so that the food is ground by the cutica gastrica. The addition of grit ingested by the bird may assist in this process. The resultant paste is then passed to the small intestine.

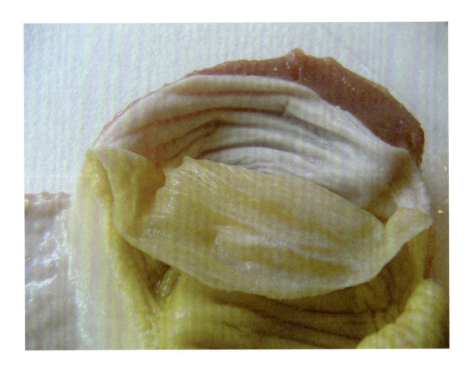

The function of the intestines is the absorption of soluble nutrients from the food and the reabsorbtion of water. The intestines are firmly fixed to the walls of the abdomen by membrane (the mesentery) and consist of an inner surface (mucosa), a secondary layer (submucosa), an inner circular layer of muscle and an outer layer of longitudinal muscle. Food moves down the intestines through the same wave action as occurs in the oesophagus. Nutrients are released by further digestion using bile and pancreatic juices and the soluble nutrients are absorbed through the intestinal wall and enter the blood circulation (portal hepatic circulation) and are carried to the liver.

The intestines are divided into regions, but these are not as distinct as in mammals, these regions being:

The **duodenum** –forms a loop around the pancreas ending where the ducts from the liver and the pancreas enter the intestine. Bile, produced in the liver, mixes with the pancreatic juices to emulsify fats, break down carbohydrates and proteins and neutralize the stomach acid. The presence of bile also stimulates the peristaltic movement of the intestines.

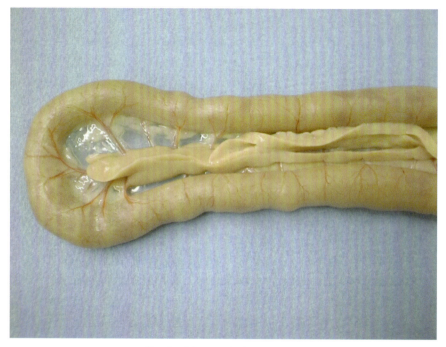

Duodenal loop enclosing pancreas

The **jejunum** – runs from the duodenum to the ileum. The junctions between the jejunum and ileum is very indistinct, but is accepted as occurring at the point where a small projection appears on the surface of the intestines. This projection, the vitelline diverticulum, denotes the point at which the yolk sac was attached to the intestines during development of the egg.

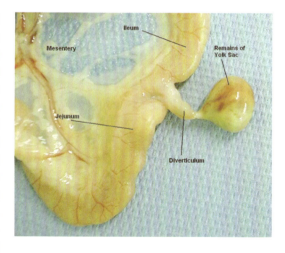

Occasionally vestigial pea-sized remains of the yolk sac can be found attached to the intestines or free within the body cavity. This occurs when the union between the yolk sac and diverticulum becomes occluded, preventing complete absorption of the yolk, which solidifies.

The **ileum** – runs from the diverticulum to the ileo-caecal junction, where the two caeca join the intestine.

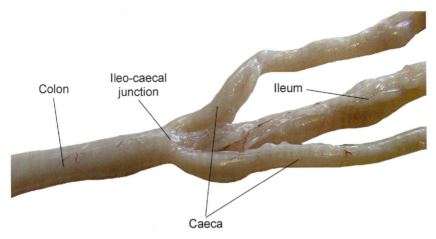

Colon | Ileo-caecal junction | Ileum | Caeca

The **caeca** are two blind-ended sacs into which portions of the intestinal contents are diverted via reverse peristalsis. The caeca empty approximately every eight hours. The caeca reabsorb water from the intestinal contents, bacteria break down cellulose, synthesize vitamins, and secrete hormones.

The **large intestine** – also known as the colon, runs from the ileo-caecal junction to the cloaca. Water is also reabsorbed in the colon.

The **cloaca** – this comprises three sections, the cuprodeum, urodeum and proctodeum. The cuprodeum joins the colon and contains faeces; the urodeum contains the openings for urine, eggs and/or sperm. The proctodeum contains the proctodeal gland and ends at the vent.

The end result of the digestive process is waste, faeces. In poultry, where water conservation is very important, the faeces tend to be dry and are capped with white uric acid crystals added as the faeces pass through the urodeum. When the caeca are emptied the droppings tend to be brown coloured and frothy and should not be confused with the constant watery droppings associated with diarrhoea.

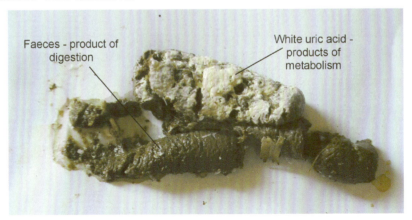

Faeces - product of digestion | White uric acid - products of metabolism

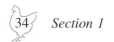

The Pancreas is an exocrine gland contained within the duodenal loop. It is a gland that secretes pancreatic juice, a solution comprising digestive enzymes and sodium bicarbonate, into the distal duodenum through 2-3 pancreatic ducts, neutralizing the acidity of the food leaving the stomach. It also performs an endocrine function, secreting insulin, which affects the metabolism of certain compounds, and glucogen that raises blood sugar levels.

THE MESENTERY

The mesentery is a membranous sheet that attaches the intestines to the abdominal cavity walls. Within the structure of the mesentery is held the various branches of the cranial mesenteric vein and artery which join to form the portal system that transports the digested nutrients to the liver.

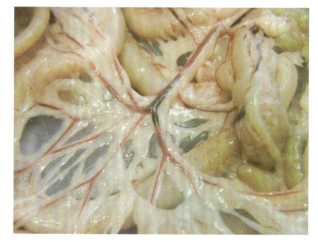

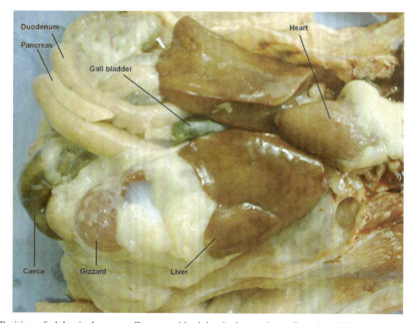

Position of abdominal organs. Carcase with abdominal covering reflected and ribcage removed

THE LIVER

GENERAL

In poultry the liver is large in proportion to the body size and occupies a large area of the abdomen. One surface of the liver is convex (parietal surface) and rests against the underside of the sternum and abdominal wall, the other (the visceral surface) is concave and lies against the spleen, gizzard, proventriculus, duodenum and jejunum. The liver consists of two lobes joined at the top by a narrow bridge or isthmus. The right lobe is marginally larger than the left (which is partially divided) and has the gall bladder, which stores bile, attached to the visceral surface.

Two tubes, (bile ducts) run from the liver to the duodenal/jejunal junction of the small intestine near the point of entry of the pancreatic ducts. One bile duct runs directly from the gall bladder (cystic duct), the other emanates from the visceral surface of the left lobe (hepatic duct). In young birds the liver is yellowish in colour due to the presence of absorbed yolk, but becomes increasingly dark brown as the bird matures.

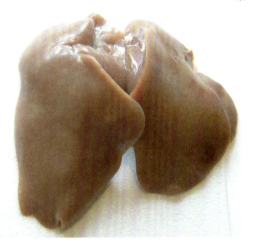

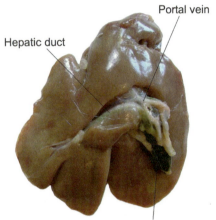

Portal vein

Hepatic duct

Gall bladder

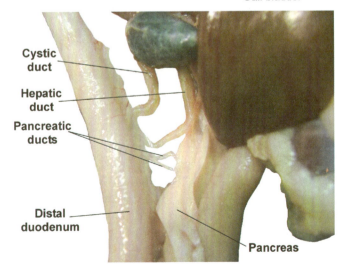

Cystic duct

Hepatic duct

Pancreatic ducts

Distal duodenum

Pancreas

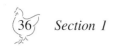

LIVER FUNCTION

The liver has many functions in the body, including:

- Production and secretion of bile, a slightly acidic solution containing two bile salts bilirubin and biliverdin, and an enzyme, amylase. As well as reducing the acidity of the intestinal contents when entering the jejunum and activating the pancreatic juices, bile emulsifies fats (reducing insoluble fats into small droplets suspended in solution enabling their absorption). Amylase speeds the breakdown reaction of carbohydrates and starch into simpler compounds.

- Filtration. The liver filters the blood; nutrients that are digested through the intestinal wall enter the hepatic portal blood circulation, by which they are carried to the liver for absorption, storage and synthesis. This filtration function also leads to the liver being the site of initial infection (primary lesions) derived from blood or intestinal sources.

- Chemical synthesis. The liver converts sugars to glycogen for storage, it breaks down fatty acids and stores them, synthesizes albumen which assists in the regulation of blood volume and produces blood clotting agents such as fibrinogen.

- Thermoregulation. The relatively large size of this organ and the chemical reactions it undertakes assists in the maintenance of an average body temperature.

RESPIRATORY SYSTEM

The purpose of the respiratory system is twofold, firstly it facilitates the exchange of oxygen between the atmosphere and the cells of the body, and secondly it allows the diffusion of carbon dioxide from the cells to the atmosphere. The cells of the body require oxygen to function; this is carried to them by the blood, carbon dioxide is produced by the cells as a waste product of their metabolism and is toxic, this is removed by the blood and exchanged for oxygen in the lungs.

In birds, this oxygen exchange is extremely efficient, vast amounts of oxygen are required to meet the physical exertion of flight, and the birds respiratory system has evolved to enable this. There are, therefore, fundamental differences in the respiratory system anatomy and function between birds and mammals.

The **lungs** are of a similar proportion to those of mammals, but have approximately 10% of the volume as they do not expand. The airflow through the lungs is one way, there are no blind-ended sacs as in mammals so consequently there is no ebb and flow of air through the lungs, it is continuous. Attached to the airways (bronchioles) of the lungs are the **airsacs**, thin, transparent bags that form part of the avian respiratory system. These airsacs (9 in poultry) cover the organs of the body and even extend into some of the long bones of the skeleton. There is no muscular diaphragm dividing the chest cavity (thorax) from the abdominal cavity, the airsacs act as bellows, drawing in air through the lungs and expelling the stale air.

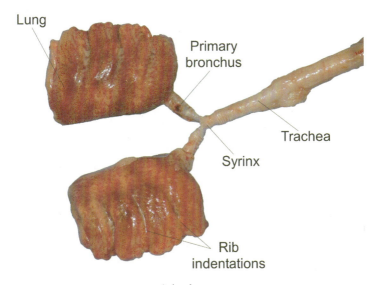

Lung

Primary bronchus

Trachea

Syrinx

Rib indentations

Avian lungs

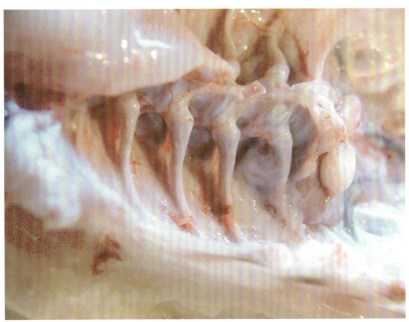

Thoracic cavity – illustrating rib arches

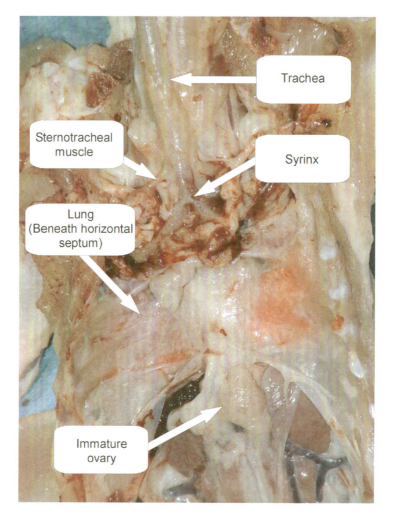

Trachea and lungs *in situ*

With the exception of the intraclavicular the airsacs are paired, two anterior thoracic, two cervical, two posterior thoracic and two abdominal.

The air travels down the trachea, through the voice box (**syrinx**) at which point the trachea splits (bifurcates) into the two main bronchi. Each bronchi constricts at the segmentum accelerans and enters the lung tissue as the **mesobronchi**; directing the air straight through to the rear airsacs (posterior thoracic and abdominal.) When these airsacs contract the air is forced back into the lungs through the **dorsobronchi** and **ventrobronchi** to the gas exchange capillaries of the **parabronchi**. The air then flows to the frontal airsacs before being exhaled.

The diagram following illustrates the airflow, the air breathed in remains in the body for two breaths.

The breathing cycle is basically:

First inhalation - Abdominal expansion draws air through to the rear air sacs.

First exhalation - Abdomen contracts forcing air through the lungs.

Second inhalation - Abdomen expands again, forcing air in lungs into forward airsacs.

Second exhalation - Abdomen contracts driving stale air out of trachea.

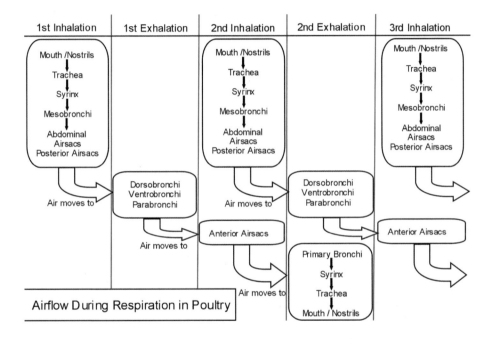

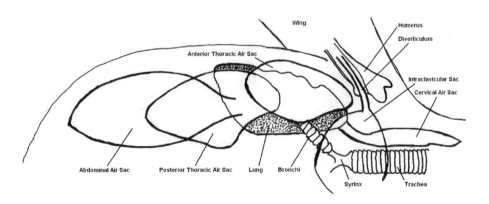

Sketch of the position of the airsacs

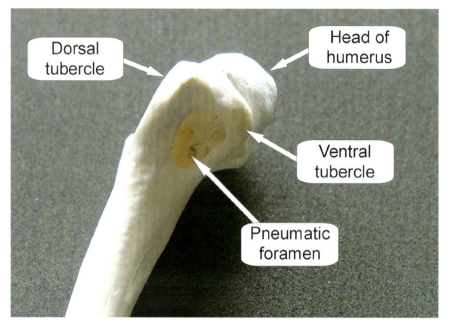

The head of the humerus – detailing the pneumatic foramen that channels the diverticulum of the intraclavicular airsac

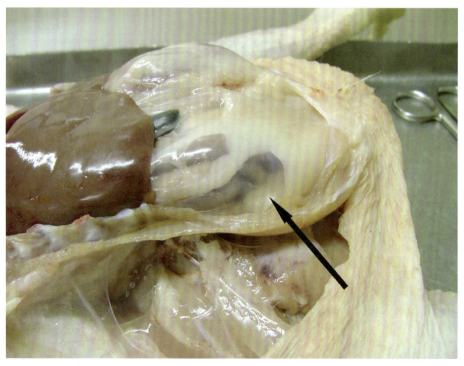

Abdominal airsac - artificially expanded

CARDIOVASCULAR SYSTEM

The cardiovascular system is a delivery system, transporting oxygen, nutrients, hormones etc to all the cells of the body to enable them to function and survive. This system also transports the waste products produced by the cells to the lungs (in the case of carbon dioxide) or to the kidneys (metabolic waste), for removal from the body, as well as redistributing heat throughout the body. The cardiovascular system consists of sealed tubes (blood vessels) containing a liquid (blood) that is circulated throughout the body by a pump (the heart).

THE HEART

In poultry the heart is conical in shape and comparatively larger than that of mammals. It is enclosed in a clear membrane sac (the pericardium) that secretes fluid to lubricate and protect the heart as it beats at a rate of 350-450 beats per minute. The heart is a muscular organ comprising four chambers, - the right atrium and ventricle and the left atrium and ventricle separated by a septum. The left side of the heart has thicker muscular walls and supplies arterial blood to the body under pressure. The ventricles are divided from the atria by valves; only the valves of the left ventricle are prevented from inverting under pressure by tendons, *Chordae tendineae*, that originate from the endocardium.

The pericardium itself has a visceral and parietal layer, the visceral pericardium being attached to the surface of the heart forming the epicardium, the parietal pericardium containing more fibrin.

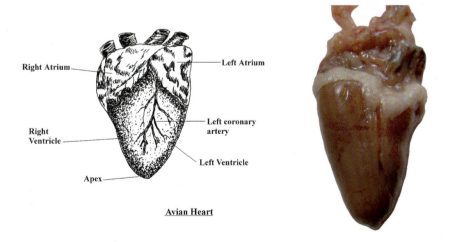

Right Atrium

Left Atrium

Right Ventricle

Left coronary artery

Left Ventricle

Apex

Avian Heart

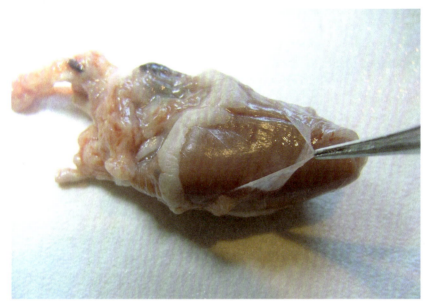

The fibrinous clear pericardium covering the heart

BLOOD VESSELS

These form a network throughout the body carrying blood to the tissues and cells, they allow fluid to escape and enter through their walls to 'bathe' the cells. There are five types of blood vessels:

Arteries	- carry oxygenated blood under pressure to
Arterioles	- smaller diameter arteries leading to
Capillaries	- very small bore vessels, some have such a small diameter the blood cells actually bend and flex to pass through them, here gas and nutrient exchange takes place.
Venuoles	- small diameter veins that take oxygen-depleted, carbon dioxide-rich blood to
Veins	- that carry the blood to the lungs for re-oxygenation

BLOOD

This is a high viscosity red fluid consisting of a fluid part (plasma) and cellular elements, that clots rapidly on exposure to air. Plasma is a straw coloured, protein rich fluid containing water, salts, nutrients, waste products of cellular metabolism and hormones. Suspended within this fluid is the cellular portion, red and white corpuscles and platelets.

The red corpuscles, erythrocytes, are nucleated in poultry and relatively inflexible in comparison with their mammalian counterparts, they possess a thin capsular membrane with extensions that enter the cell forming a fine internal lattice, and are distinctive in that they possess no nucleus. The membranous lattice enmeshes haemoglobin, a protein that readily converts to oxyhaemoglobin in the presence of oxygen in the lungs and transports this oxygen to the cell tissues where it is released in return for the carbon dioxide waste of the cells which binds to the haemoglobin until returned to the lungs.

The white corpuscles, leucocytes, form part of the immune system recognising and digesting foreign material (including bacteria), neutralising toxins and removing dead or damaged tissue. The platelets possess no nucleus and form part of the clotting mechanism.

BLOOD VESSELS

The blood vessels carry the blood throughout the body, arteries carrying blood under pressure from the heart, veins carrying blood back to the heart. The arteries have a three layered wall, an inner wall (*tunica interna*) of endothelial cells on an elastic connective tissue membrane, a central layer (*tunica media*) comprised of smooth muscle and elastic tissue, and a fibrous outer layer (*tunica adventitia*) that provides a defence against overexpansion of the arterial wall and possible rupture. This layering allows for expansion of the artery during the pump phase of the hearts movement (systole) followed by elastic relaxation and return to normal size during the rest phase, an action which also serves to further propel the blood along the artery. The arteries branch to smaller diameter arterioles which in turn branch into capillaries from which they are differentiated by retaining a proportion of muscle in their walls to regulate blood flow. The capillaries are thin tubes of endothelial cells on a thin connective tissue support, allowing fluid to leave the blood at the arterial end of the capillary bed to 'bathe' the tissue cells before a percentage of this fluid re-enters toward the venous portion of the capillary bed. The capillaries then reform into venuoles and then veins for return to the heart. The veins are thinner walled than arteries as they do not suffer the effects of the systolic 'pump', the muscular *tunica media* being confined to the larger veins. The *tunica interna* is thinner but forms one way valves within the vein to prevent back flow of the low pressure blood.

BLOOD CIRCULATION

The circulation of the blood throughout the body can be subdivided into three stages or circuits, the pulmonary circulation, the systemic circulation and the portal circulation.

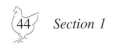

PULMONARY CIRCULATION

This system provides for the reoxygenation of the blood. Blood is pumped from the right ventricle via the pulmonary artery which bifurcates to enter each side of the lungs where further subdivision of the arteries to arterioles and capillaries occurs. Once gaseous exchange takes place the pulmonary capillaries unite to form veins to take the purified blood back to the left auricle of the heart. Increased blood pressure within this system is common and can lead to systemic disturbance (see ascites).

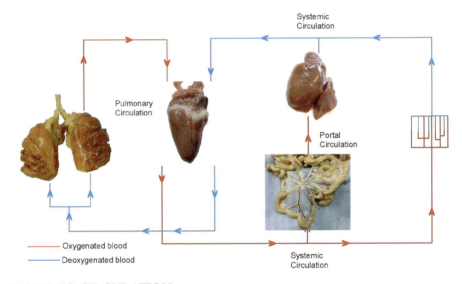

Systemic
Circulation

Pulmonary
Circulation

Portal
Circulation

———— Oxygenated blood
———— Deoxygenated blood

Systemic
Circulation

SYSTEMIC CIRCULATION

The oxygenated blood then passes from the left auricle to the left ventricle via the bicuspid valve and is pumped through the aorta from which arteries branch off followed by further subdivision into arterioles and capillaries conveying the blood to all the tissues of the body. These capillaries then reunite to form venuoles and veins which carry the impure deoxygenated blood back to the heart via the anterior and posterior vena cava.

PORTAL CIRCULATION

The portal circulation carries the blood from the intestines and stomachs to the liver via the portal vein. Once the blood has passed through the liver and the nutrients removed for conversion or added to the blood by the liver it passes into the normal circulation by being discharged into the posterior vena cava or via the hepatic vein back to the heart.

BLOOD CLOTTING

The clotting of blood is achieved by the action of platelets in conjunction with the protein fibrinogen which is carried in the plasma. On exposure to air, platelets bind together and release thrombokinase. Thrombokinase reacts with prothrombin, produced by the liver, and plasma calcium to produce the enzyme thrombin which then converts fibrinogen to fibrin. The filamentous fibrin then forms a lattice of insoluble material that enmeshes corpuscles to form a clot. Blood serum is plasma from which fibrinogen has been removed during clotting.

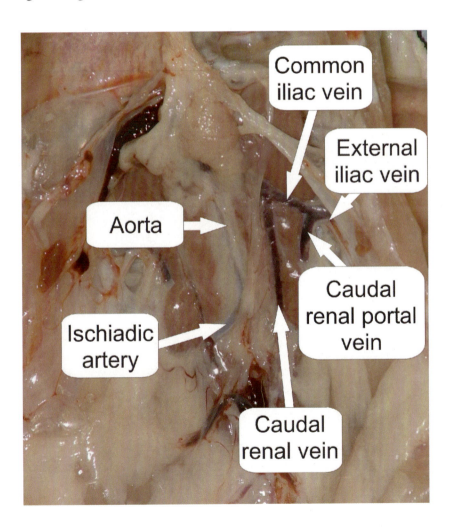

Visible blood vessels in the vicinity of the kidneys

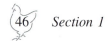

UROGENITAL SYSTEM

KIDNEYS

The kidneys of poultry are situated in recesses either side of the vertebral column on the underside of the synsacrum. Each kidney is divided into three lobes, the anterior, middle and posterior. The function of the kidneys is filtration; blood enters the kidneys via the renal artery and renal portal veins where impurities and the products of cell metabolism are removed. The kidneys also maintain the water balance of the body. Nitrogen based impurities are excreted by the kidneys as uric acid (unlike the urea excreted by mammalian kidneys.) This urate is water-soluble and in its dilute form (a cream coloured viscous fluid) it is passed down the ureters originating in the middle lobe. There is no bladder in poultry; the ureters pass directly to the urodeum of the cloaca. There, further water is reabsorbed from the urate, which is then passed as a whitish crystalline deposit with the faeces.

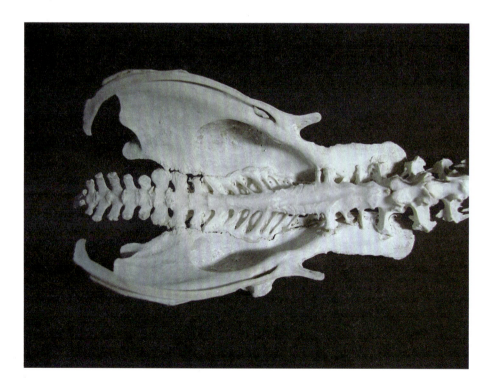

Interior of the pelvis, illustrating the cavities occupied by the kidneys

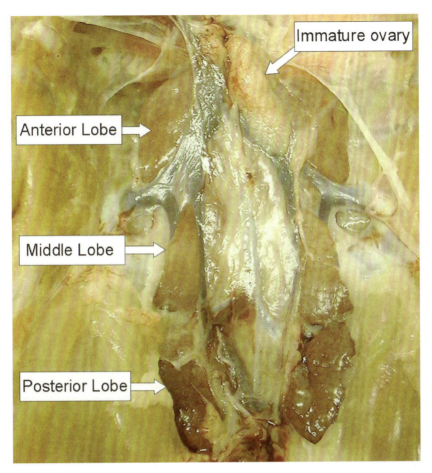

The kidneys in an immature female

FEMALE REPRODUCTIVE SYSTEM

In poultry only the left ovary is functional, the right ovary degenerates soon after hatching, the left ovary is found to one side of the anterior lobe of the left kidney. The ovary is a mass of cyst-like ova, ranging in size and colour, starting as small, white spheres but becoming increasingly larger (2-3cm in diameter) and yellow as they mature. When mature the ripened ova is released and collected by the oviduct, a tube containing glands that form the egg proper and deliver it to the cloaca for laying. The oviduct is formed by five indistinct sections, the time taken for the ova to be collected, form into an egg and enter the cloaca is approximately 24 hours.

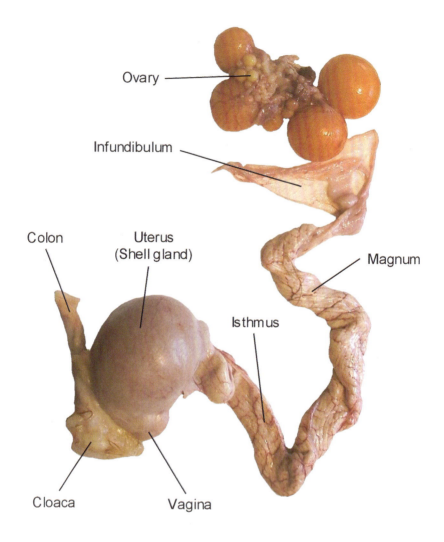

Sections of the oviduct

Section name	Approx length	Duration of ova passage	Function
Infundibulum	10cm	18 minutes	Collects ova from ovary
Magnum	35cm	3 hours	Albumen (egg white) secreted
Isthmus	10cm	1.25 hours	Shell membrane formed
Uterus	10cm	20 hours	Hard shell formed
Vagina	8cm		Transfers egg to cloaca

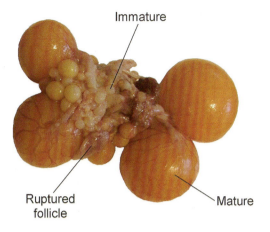

A mature ovary

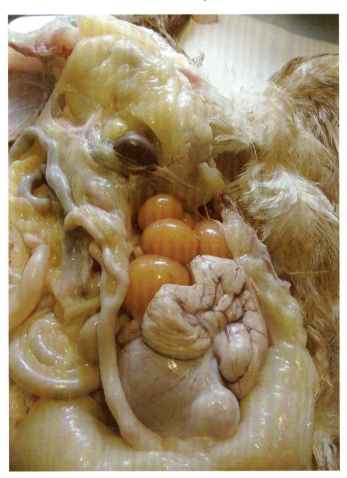

Female reproductive system in situ – Sternum removed and digestive system laterally transposed

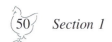

MALE REPRODUCTIVE SYSTEM

The testes are paired, yellowish-cream coloured, oval structures situated near the anterior lobe of the kidney. These enlarge during the breeding season. Semen is discharged down two deferent ducts that spiral down the body next to the two ureters and discharge into the urodeum of the cloaca.

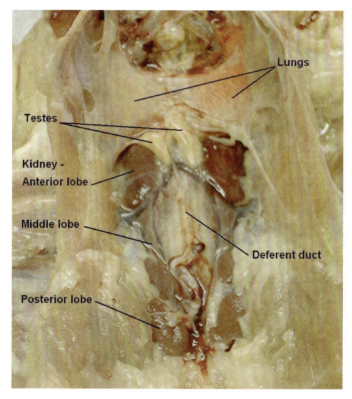

Immature male reproductive system in situ

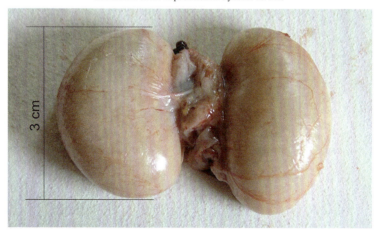

Mature testicles – broiler breeder

IMMUNE SYSTEM

Organs of the body considered to be part of the immune system include the cloacal bursa, caecal tonsils, spleen, and **thymus** which is seen as 6-8 pink, flattened lobes running down either side of the neck near the jugular vein. As well as hormone secretion (see Endocrine glands section), it is in the thymus that the T-cells are matured and released (See Immunity in section 2 - Diseases of Poultry).

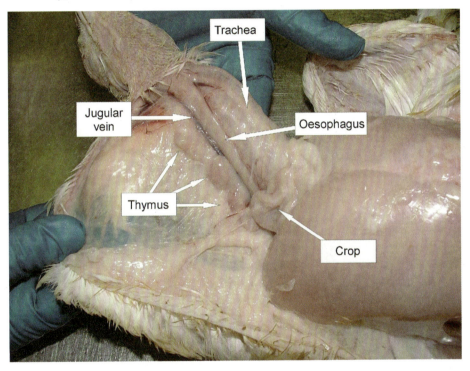

Superficial dissection of the neck

B-cells are matured in the **cloacal bursa (Bursa of Fabricius)** that is formed from, and opens into, the proctodeum of the cloaca. The bursa is a round structure found above the rear of the cloaca, between the cloaca and the caudal vertebrae. It ceases to mature B-cells after 14-16 weeks after which it begins to waste away (atrophy). The loss of production of B-cells and hence the humoral immunity before this time, due to disease such as Gumboro (Infectious Bursal Disease) produces an immune deficiency syndrome and the bird becomes susceptible to further diseases. This has earned Gumboro the unofficial title of "chicken AIDS".

Cross Section of the Cloaca.
Left Side.

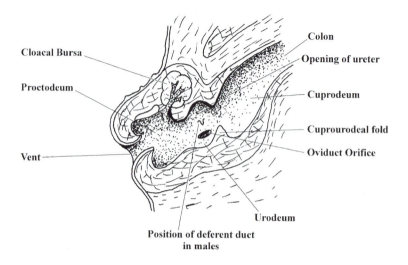

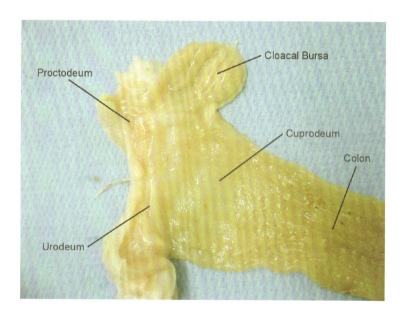

The **spleen** is a spherical, bright red organ situated near the liver. It contains
a mixture of red and white pulp although this demarcation is more discrete
than in mammals; the white pulp includes macrophages, large phagocytes
that in the spleen have the specific function of removing diseased or old

blood cells. These red blood cells lose their flexibility when in this condition and become trapped when the blood passes through the spleen. The trapped cells are digested by the macrophages and their constituents are recycled.

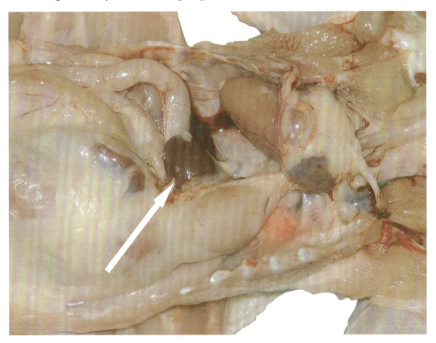

The position of the spleen, liver removed

LYMPHOID TISSUE

This tissue, also known as peripheral lymphoid tissue, forms part of the Avian Lymphatic system. This system operates in conjunction with the blood circulation, and consists of a fluid, lymph, that 'bathes' the cells of the body, lymphatic vessels and peripheral lymphoid tissue.

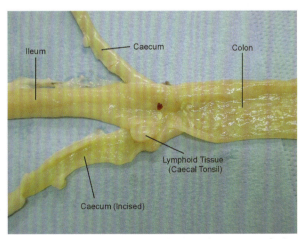

Lymph originates as part of the blood plasma; it leaches out of the capillaries and bathes the cells of tissues, one of its functions being the transportation of nutrients to the cells and the removal of metabolic products from them. It is a slightly yellow, transparent fluid comprising mostly water,

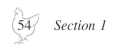

the remainder being composed of plasma proteins and other chemical substances. It also carries lymphocytes, the white blood cells responsible for part of the immune defence of the body. Lymph is collected from these tissues and enters lymph vessels that run either side of the blood vessels. These vessels combine at two large lymphatic ducts, which then discharge the lymph back into the bloodstream in the area of the jugular vein.

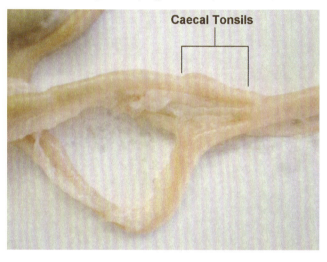

Caecal Tonsils

Situated along the lymphatic vessels are areas of peripheral lymphoid tissue, a latticework of tissue that contains lymphocytes in its interspaces, these form the avian equivalent of the enclosed lymph nodes of mammals. Lymphoid tissue is found in nearly all the internal organs, but is not obvious as it is not encapsulated and blends in with surrounding tissue, it is evident, however, at the junction of the ileum and caeca at the '**caecal tonsils**'.

Lymphoid tissue filters out and destroys noxious agents, such as bacteria, as part of its immune function; this leads to inflammation of the tissue rendering it visible to the naked eye. This is particularly the case in certain disease conditions such as Duck Viral Enteritis, where a characteristic lesion is the visible, enlarged annular bands and discs of lymphoid tissue called Peyer's patches present in the mucosa and submucosal tissues of the intestines, especially the ileum.

NERVOUS SYSTEM

INTRODUCTION

The nervous system is the body's messenger system, nerves prompting activities such as muscular action, organ activity and hormone secretion, as well as informing the brain of the condition of the body systems and the environment. The nervous system is divided into two regions, the Central Nervous System (the brain and spinal cord) and the Peripheral Nervous System (organs, muscles, skin etc.) These systems themselves function on two levels, the somatic nervous system, co-coordinating impulses that are under conscious control, and the autonomic system, controlling involuntary action such as heart beat, organ function and hormone secretion by glands.

NERVES

Nerves are non-microscopic, string like structures formed by bundled nerve cells that pass impulses between the central nervous system and parts or organs of the body. There are three basic forms of nerve, categorized by their function and the direction of the impulses, either from the central nervous system, to the central nervous system or both ways, these nerve types being efferent, sensory and intermediate. Efferent nerves (also known as motor nerves) transmit impulses from the central nervous system usually to groups of muscles; Sensory nerves convey impulses such as temperature or pain to the central nervous system and Intermediate nerves transmit impulses both ways.

NERVE CELLS

The nerve cell or neuron is the basis of the nervous system. The cell body is surrounded by dendrites, extensions of the cell wall, of which one is elongated to form the axon. During neuron development the axon is surrounded by specialist cell (Schwann cells) that spiral around the axon, this envelope of cells then secretes a layer of myelin forming an insulating sheath. Bundles of axons form the nerves; the sciatic nerve serving the hind leg contains axons of over a metre in length. The nerve chain forms circuits throughout the body, the cellular electrical impulse travelling along the axon from one nerve cell to the dendrite of another. Each nerve cell is separated from the next by a junction gap (synapse) across which chemical transmitters cross causing cellular excitement and a continuation of the impulse.

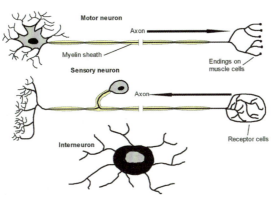

CENTRAL NERVOUS SYSTEM

The **brain** is situated in the cranial cavity of the skull. As in mammals it consists of two pear shaped hemispheres comprising the cerebrum and cerebellum. The brain is relatively smaller than in mammals and is smoother; however, the area dealing with the processing of information from the optic nerves is extremely well developed by comparison to mammals, affording the bird better eyesight and visual clarity. The base of the brain forms the medulla oblongata.

The **spinal cord** originates from the medulla oblongata and runs through a channel formed by the hollow mid-section of the spinal vertebrae down to the last free vertebrae of the tail.

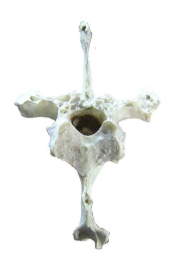

Thoracic vertebra

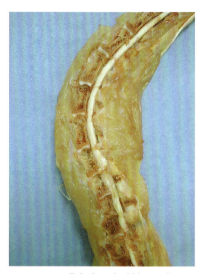

Spinal cord within canal

PERIPHERAL NERVOUS SYSTEM

The peripheral nerves emanate symmetrically from each side of the spinal cord and pass through the body of the vertebrae. The nerves can be single or grouped together (plexus or ganglia). Two major groups of nerves are important in meat inspection, the brachial plexus with nerves branching out to the pectoral muscles and the wings which originates from the last four cervical and first thoracic vertebrae, and the

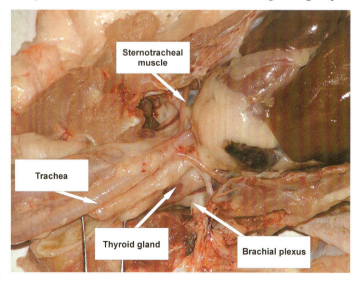

sciatic or ischiadic nerve, the widest nerve in the body, which branches from the lumbrosacral plexus and runs down the thigh.

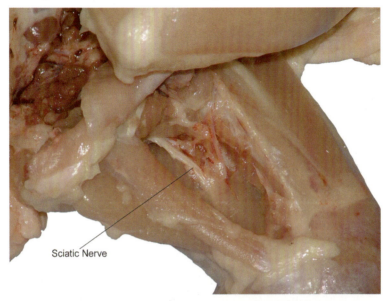

Position of sciatic nerve, overlying musculature removed

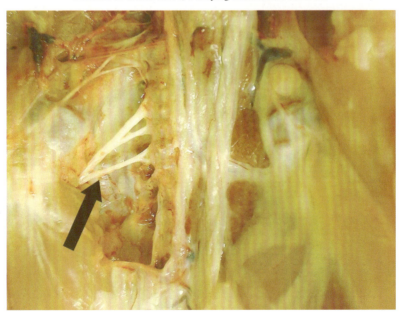

Lumbosacral plexus – revealed by blunt dissection of the kidney

Normally these nerves are white with feint bands, but when infected by diseases such as Marek's Disease, become thickened which affects their ability to send and receive stimuli, resulting in paralysis of the part of the anatomy they supply. This is true of any part of the nervous system, affections of the spinal cord can paralyze the body from that point down, as can occur in conditions such as spondylolisthesis.

ENDOCRINE SYSTEM

Defined as the ductless glands, organs of the endocrine system possess specialist cells that secrete hormones - chemical transmitters used for communication and control within the body. These glands include the pituitary, thyroid, parathyroid, thymus, adrenals, pancreas and gonads.

THYROID GLAND

These are paired oval brownish glands located cranially to the crop at the thoracic inlet close to the brachial plexus. They are composed of densely packed sacs containing a clear viscose fluid.

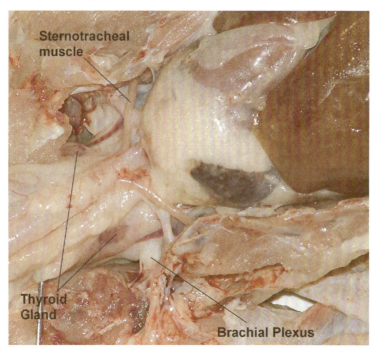

PARATHYROID GLAND

These are two to three small glands situated cranially to the thyroid glands.

PITUITARY GLAND (HYPOPHYSIS)

This small yellowish-brown bi-lobed gland is situated in a protective hollow in the cranium on the midline of the ventral brain. The action of the anterior and posterior lobes is controlled by the hypothalamus from which the pituitary is separated by a small portal system of blood vessels by which communication between the two organs is achieved.

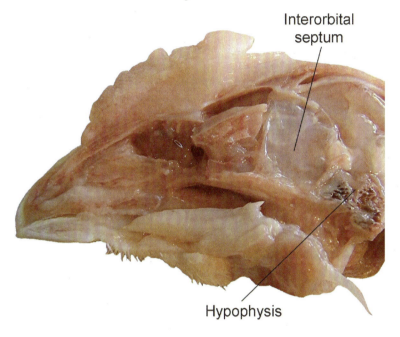

Position of the hypophysis

THYMUS

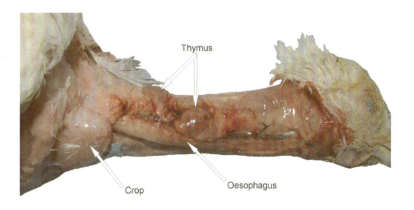

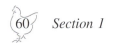
The thymus glands are located in the neck and are associated with the jugular veins. These glands are primarily responsible for the maturation of stem cells into T-lymphocytes and regress at sexual maturity.

ADRENAL GLANDS

These are paired brown triangular shaped glands approximately 1cm in length found cranial to the anterior lobe of the kidneys. Each adrenal gland is composed of two differing tissues with different functions and consists of a cortex surrounding a medulla.

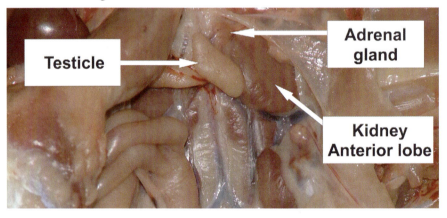

PANCREAS

In addition to the exocrine function of the pancreas in the digestive process a second endocrine function, described in the following table, is undertaken by foci of specialist cells (Islets of Langerhans) found throughout the substance of the pancreas.

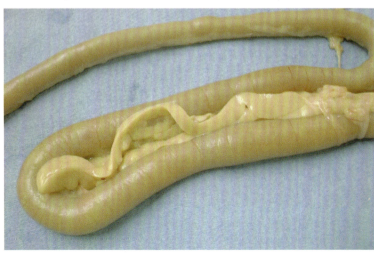

ENDOCRINE GLANDS – SUMMARY OF FUNCTION

Thymus   Development and maturation of T-lymphocytes. Also sexual development.

Adrenal Cortex   Produces multiple hormones (corticoids) which maintain blood volume, have an anti-inflammatory action, maintenance of blood glucose levels and fat deposition. Secretion controlled by anterior pituitary gland.

Adrenal Medulla   Secretes adrenalin and noradrenalin for stimulation of cardio-respiratory system, increase in blood sugar levels and increased metabolic rate. Also raises blood pressure by vaso-constriction.

Pancreas   Insulin and glucagon work antagonistically to maintain blood sugar levels, insulin prompting conversion and storage of glucose in liver and muscles, glucagon prompting release.

Thyroid   Regulates metabolic rate through production of thyroxin prompted by hormone released by anterior pituitary in response to monitoring by the hypothalamus. Also produces calcitonin to maintain constant blood calcium levels.

Parathyroid   Secretes parathyroid hormone influencing calcium to be absorbed into bone from blood. Works antagonistically with calcitonin.

Pituitary Anterior   Produces many hormones, primarily TSH (Thyroid stimulating hormone) in response to messages from the hypothalamus.

DISEASES OF POULTRY

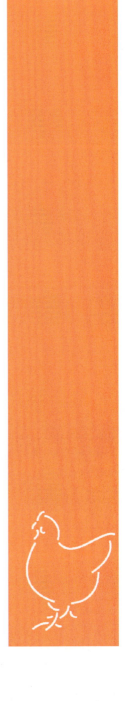

INTRODUCTION

The survival of an animal depends on the symbiotic function of all the bodily systems. Disease can be considered to be an abnormality in the structure or function of these systems, and even an inability of the animal to perform as expected in relation to its peers. The traditional concept of disease is that there is a causal factor that produces recognisable macroscopic and microscopic lesions that can lead to identification of the causal factor. In this section infectious diseases are considered, including those due to viral, bacterial and fungal pathogens, be they of communicable origin (passed from one animal to another) or commensal organisms (organisms that form part of the normal microflora associated with the animal).

The role of the Meat Inspector is to determine whether the carcase or part carcase is fit for human consumption, given the macroscopic evidence of lesions presented.

Of greatest importance are zoonotic diseases, those that are naturally transmissible between vertebrate animals and man, such as anthrax, brucellosis.

ROUTES OF INFECTION

Inhalation – The causative agents are drawn into the body during the act of inspiration. Tuberculosis lesions usually have primary foci within the lung tissue. Other respiratory infections in poultry tend to be devastating due to both the rearing conditions and the respiratory anatomy of the bird.

Ingestion- Infection and subsequent spread is achieved by entry of the infectious agent via the digestive tract, initial lesions in this tract are usually followed by transference of the infection to the liver via the hepatic portal blood circulation. This infection route also includes migration of commensal intestinal flora or their proliferation should the intestinal conditions change to suit them.

Inoculation – Penetration of the physical barrier to infection, provided by the skin and mucous membranes, allows entry of micro organisms, either through exposure of subcutaneous tissue to environmental contamination or by the injection of these agents that may be present on or in the object penetrating the barrier as occurs in wounds. Both intensively reared and free-range poultry can clamber over each other and scratch the surface of the skin. Other vices can also occur, including feather pecking and cannibalism which can introduce infection.

Congenital- Vertical transmission from the mother to the offspring, if this infection occurs before the foetus has developed its own immune system (before third trimester) any infectious organism can be included in the phase where recognition of 'self' occurs so that any infection may not be countered

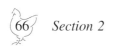

as it is not recognised as foreign material. Infection acquired in utero, both during the shell formation stage and through the porous shell itself, can occur.

The initial site of microscopic or macroscopic infection is known as the primary focus. The description of condition being a peracute infection indicates rapid onset (few hours), an acute infection generally denotes one of short duration (1-2 days) as opposed to a chronic infection (1 week plus.)

IMMUNITY

Immunity can be described as non-susceptibility to a particular disease, or the pathogenic effects of micro organisms, or chemical toxins. Immunity is the ability of the body to distinguish foreign material and to neutralize or eliminate it. This is achieved through the body's immune response. Foreign material which can be toxins, foreign proteins and even parts of the polysaccharide cell walls of bacteria and other tissue, is recognised by the presence of substances called antigens. The immunity of a body to infection, either exogenous (where external organisms breach the body defences) or endogenous (where natural flora become pathogenic), is dependant on the inter-reaction of three lines of defence. The first two lines of defence, the skin/mucous membranes and the cellular/humoral factors are innate and non-specific; they are a normal part of the body and react to the presence of any foreign body. The third line of defence, the acquired immune response, is specific to each individual type of invading micro organism and takes longer to mobilise. The first lines of defence form the initial immune reaction and initiate the specific response.

SKIN/ MUCOUS MEMBRANES

These form the initial defence to infection in three ways. Firstly they provide a physical barrier, which produces antimicrobial factors such as the fatty acids present in sweat, the lysosomes in mucous, and surfactant in the lungs. Secondly the mucous membranes provide a mechanical defence, wave-like movement of hair-like projections called cilia of the cells in conjunction with mucous remove foreign particles. Thirdly the presence of normal flora, known as commensal organisms, on the skin and mucous membranes compete with pathogens for space and nutrients, this competition normally involving the production of short chain fatty acids that act as microbial agents against the invading organisms.

CELLULAR FACTORS

Specialised cells (collectively known as phagocytes) free within the body systems are capable of **phagocytosis**, literally the eating of cells; these include neutrophils which primarily attack extracellular bacteria, eosinophils which attack parasites and macrophages that attack intracellular bacteria, protozoa and viruses. The process of phagocytosis is four staged, beginning with **chemotaxis**, whereby the phagocyte is attracted to the invader by chemicals produced by the invader itself as well as the body due to the presence of the invader. The second stage is the **adhesion** of the phagocyte to the invader. This is usually accomplished by the phagocyte extending its membrane wall into a 'false limb' (pseudopodium) that reaches out and attaches to the invader. The invader is then **ingested**; the pseudopodium retracts, drawing the invader into the phagocyte, which then extends further pseudopodia around the organism trapping it in a space called a vacuole within the phagocyte. The final stage is the **killing** of the invader, this is achieved either though an oxidative burst by chemicals such as hydrogen peroxide, or through the damaging of the bacterial membrane by lysosomes present in the phagocyte. Enzymes then degrade the dead bacterium.

HUMORAL FACTORS

These assist the process of phagocytosis and are a chain of chemical reactions of serum proteins, the product of one reaction being the catalyst or initiator of the next. The products of these reactions induce chemotaxis, aid adhesion of the phagocyte, lyse (kill) organisms by breaking down the cell wall and increase the vascular permeability allowing the increased supply of phagocytes to the infected area.

ACQUIRED IMMUNE RESPONSE

This specific immune defence is acquired after exposure to infection, and forms the basis of the theory of vaccination. It relies on **antibodies**, molecules of immunoglobulins that comprise three areas, two constant that activate phagocytes and humoral responses and a third that 'keys' onto the specific antigen of the invading organism. Each microbe is therefore recognised by a specific antibody that attaches to it, attracts phagocytes and triggers the humoral factors. The acquired immune response is dependant on cells known as **lymphocytes**, of which there are two groups, characterised by their function and site of maturity. Lymphocytes are derived from stem cells that travel to areas of the body to mature. **B-cells** are antibody producing cells that are matured in the bone marrow in mammals and the cloacal bursa in poultry, **T-cells** are matured and released from the thymus and are involved in cell mediated immunity and assisting the production of antibodies in B-cells.

Each B-cell produces one specific type of antibody and carries large numbers of these on its surface to act as receptors. When confronted with the infectious agent that displays the specific antigen that allows the receptors to lock, the B-cell is activated, multiplies and stimulates other plasma cells to produce copies of the antibody, producing large numbers of cloned B-cells called **affector cells**. Once the infection has been overcome, some of these B-cells remain viable as '**memory cells**' and remain present should the infectious agent be encountered in the future.

T-cells have various functions, but are primarily aimed at intracellular microbes. **Cytotoxic** T-cells recognise the antigen in virus-infected cells and kill the cell before the virus is released and also produces chemicals that create resistance to infection in neighbouring cells. **Suppressor** T-cells decrease the activity of other T and B-cells. **Helper/inducer** T-cells assist other T-cells to become cytotoxic, help B-cells produce antibodies, recognise microbial antigens in phagocytes and produce a chemical to activate the macrophage to kill the microbe.

Inflammation is a localised response to tissue damage or the presence of antigens. The local capillaries enlarge and increase permeability allowing large numbers of lymphocytes and phagocytes to enter the area, which then proceed to localise and neutralise the cause of the inflammatory response. The classic signs of inflammation are side effects of these changes and include heat, pain, swelling, redness and disturbance of function. Once the causal factor has been overcome, the result to the affected tissue can be regeneration, scarring or cell death (necrosis).

There are various forms of inflammation including those leading to the formation of fibrous tissue (fibrinous inflammation), promoting adhesion of adjacent organs or membranes (adhesive inflammation) and diphtheric inflammation, where fibrinous exudates are formed firmly attached to underlying tissue such as occurs in cases of necrotic enteritis.

In poultry the inflammatory reaction tends to be rapid with the deposition of fibrin being predominant.

BACTERIA

SIZE AND STRUCTURE

Bacteria are single celled organisms classed as prokaryotic organisms, with varying shapes (morphologies) including spherical, rod shaped, comma shaped, spiral and ranging in size from approximately 0.5-6.0ìm.

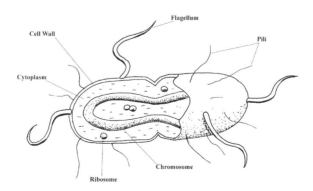

Prokaryotic organisms (bacteria and green celled algae) are distinguished from other living organisms by containing DNA in a double stranded loop (that is unenclosed by a nuclear membrane), small ribosomes (granules containing RNA) and no endoplasmic reticulum (a network of membranes within a cell involved in protein, lipid and glycogen synthesis). They are also characterised by the absence of mitochondria or other membrane enclosed organelles, and the possession of a complex protein cell wall (with the exception of mycoplasma.)

The bacterial cell structure includes a rigid cell wall and in many bacteria a mucoid polysaccharide layer complements this. This capsule resists absorption and destruction (phagocytosis) by white blood cells and also aids adherence to tissues.

The pili (fimbrae) are hair-like in appearance, can aid attachment to host cells, are anti-phagocytic and can avoid host antibody response by rapidly altering their antigenic protein, pilin.

Flagella are much longer than pili and provide mobility for the bacterium. The bacteria can have one flagellum at one or both ends (monotrichous), many flagella at one or both ends (lopotrichous), or be 'covered with hair' (peritrichous). Mobility is achieved by clockwise or counter clockwise rotation of the flagella.

Certain bacteria have the ability to sporulate (e.g. *Clostridium* and *Bacillus* spp.), where an extremely tough protective coat surrounds concentrated bacterial DNA. The cell becomes metabolically inert and can survive dehydration, heat and most chemical agents for years, until favourable conditions for growth reactivate the bacterium.

ENERGY, NUTRITION AND GROWTH

Bacteria use three sources for their energy requirements, light (phototrophy), chemical reactions (chemotrophy) or a host cell (paratrophy).

Nutritionally bacteria can be divided into two types. Autotrophs, which can synthesise nutrients from inorganic raw materials, and heterotrophs, which depend on preformed organic molecules from the environment as the source of nutrients, and can only survive intracellularly, they possess DNA and RNA but only have a certain amount of metabolic activity.

Bacterial growth is by binary fission, where the internal contents of the bacterium halve, split and then reform into two matching bacterium, the doubling time varying from 20 minutes (*E.coli*) to 24 hours (tubercle bacilli). The process of binary fission means that one bacterium becomes two, two become four, four become eight, and eight become sixteen and so on. Given balanced growth, where all required nutrients are available, the growth curve of bacteria follows distinct phases. After an initial lag phase, high-virulence exponential growth occurs during the log phase, followed by a stationary phase where the number of bacteria produced is equal to the number dying, which is in turn followed by the decline phase where the number dying is greater than the number produced as the available nutrients are used up.

Each bacterial species has varying requirements for optimum growth, including available nutrients, temperature, available moisture in the form of water activity (Aw), and the pH or hydrogen ion concentration of their growth medium.

Taking these factors in order, bacterial growth requires water-soluble nutrients, and high protein foods are favoured such as eggs, fish and meat. Food was historically salted to preserve it, which reduces moisture as well as preventing the osmotic diffusion of nutrients into bacterial cells.

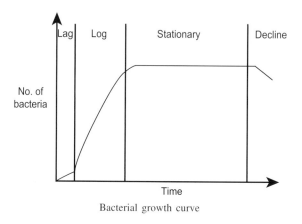

Bacterial growth curve

In terms of temperature, the lower the temperature, the slower bacteria grow. Most disease causing bacteria (pathogens) cannot grow below 4°C and none can grow below 0°C, spoilage bacteria can grow at temperatures down to -5°C. As these are the only two groups of bacteria present on meat, at temperatures below -5°C all bacterial growth ceases.

Each bacterial species has an optimum temperature for growth, as well as a temperature range in which they grow, it is generally accepted that there are four groups:

	Optimum	Range	
Psychrophiles	Below 20°C	-5 to 25°C	Includes spoilage bacteria prevalent in cold stores and refrigerators
Psychrotrophs	Above 20°C	-5 to 40°C	
Mesophiles	20 to 45°C	10 to 56°C	Includes most common pathogens such as *E.coli*, *Staphylococcus aureus* and *Campylobacter jejuni*
Thermophiles	Above 45°C	35 to 80°C	Important in canning

The moisture content, or available water level (Aw), is vital to the growth of bacteria. Pure water has an Aw value of 1.0. Bacteria have a preferred optimum available water value of around 0.99, however, *Staphylococcus aureus* will grow at 0.89 and some bacteria will grow as low as 0.75.

The hydrogen ion concentration, or pH, of the medium also affects bacterial growth. Water has a neutral ph of 7, pH values from 1 to 7 are decreasingly acidic (decreasing concentration of +H ions) and those from 7 to 14 are increasingly alkaline, (increasing concentration of –OH ions). Bacteria prefer mediums with a pH of around 7; most bacteria will not grow in food with a pH below 4.5.

TOXINS

Bacteria possess the ability to form toxins, chemicals that alter the characteristic of cells and tissue, both for the purpose of defence against attack, and to increase the invasive potential of the bacteria. There are two types of toxin, endotoxin and exotoxin.

Endotoxins are released into surrounding tissue only when the bacterium breaks down, produced from polyliposaccharides that form part of the cell wall. Exotoxins are formed from proteins and are excreted from the bacterium into surrounding tissues. Bacterial Exotoxins, such as that produced by *Clostridium botulinum* (botulism) are the most potent poisons known to man.

BACTERIAL IDENTIFICATION

In general, owing to secondary infection and the fact that various bacteria can manifest themselves in similar lesions in the affected organism, identification of the infectious agent is conducted in laboratories by culturing samples.

Bacteria are classified in various ways including their shape/size, motility, resistance to antibiotics, oxygen requirements, culture media etc. One of the identifying tests conducted is Gram's staining in which the bacteria are initially stained with crystal violet, treated with iodine solution and then decolourised with alcohol. When observed under a microscope the bacterial cells either retain a deep purple colouration and are said to be Gram positive, or their complex cell wall chemical structure resists iodine and the walls are decolourised by the alcohol and are said to be Gram negative.

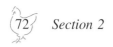

VIRUSES

Viruses are obligate parasites, they do not contain the biochemical mechanisms for their own replication and are unable to replicate outside of a living cell.

The basic viral particle (nucleocapsid) consists of linear genetic material (DNA or RNA) surrounded by a protein coat (capsid) composed of capsomeres. Some viruses are also enclosed in a membranous envelope of lipoprotein; in the case of the influenza virus this coat is formed from the host's cellular tissue and inhibits the body's auto immune response.

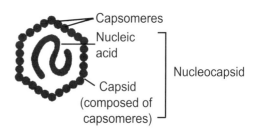

A virion is the complete viral particle, found extracellularly and capable of surviving in a metabolically inert form and possessing the ability to infect living cells. Virion range in size from 0.003 to 0.05 µm.

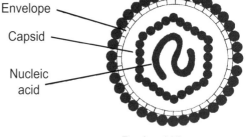

Enveloped Virus

Viruses replicate by using the biochemical mechanisms of a host cell to synthesize and assemble their separate components. When attached to a host cell, only the viral nucleic acid and in some cases a few enzymes, are injected into the cell. The nucleic acid is then replicated within the cell, followed by the synthesis of the capsid.

After infection by a virus, there are four possible effects on the host cell.

• Transformation of normal cells to tumour cells. Followed by division and the production of a tumour.

• Lytic infection. After viral multiplication the cell dies releasing the virus.

• Persistent Infection. After viral multiplication there is a slow release of the virus without cell death.

• Latent Infection. After viral multiplication the virus is present in the cell but not causing harm. Later emerges in lytic infection.

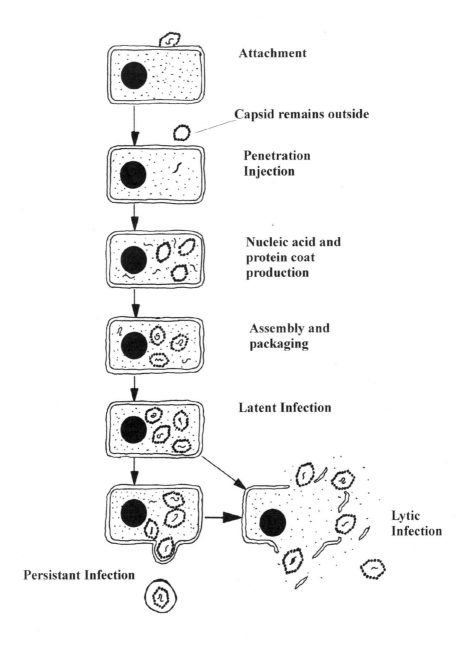

Attachment

Capsid remains outside

Penetration Injection

Nucleic acid and protein coat production

Assembly and packaging

Latent Infection

Persistant Infection

Lytic Infection

Replication cycle of a virus

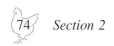

VIRUS TYPES

Adenovirus	Unenveloped, linear, double stranded nucleic acid.
Birnavirus	Unenveloped. (Bi=two) double stranded RNA present in two segments.
Coronavirus	Enveloped. Corona refers to the crown-like appearance of spikes on the envelope. A cytocidal, organ specific virus leading to progressive degeneration.
Herpesvirus	Enveloped. Large, double stranded linear DNA, icosahedral capsid.
Orthomyxovirus	Enveloped. Influenza virus. Type A affects humans and animals, Types B&C affect only humans. RNA genome divided into eight RNA molecules.
Paramyxovirus	Enveloped. Infective mechanism relies on fusion of the envelope with the host cell membrane. RNA protected by helical nucleocapsid.
Parvovirus	Unenveloped. Smallest and simplest viral particle. Icosahedral capsule containing one molecule of single stranded DNA.
Picornavirus	Unenveloped. Pico-RNA literally means small RNA that is single stranded.
Pox virus	Large ovoid or brick shaped viruses, replicates in the cytoplasm of cells. First virus to be seen microscopically.

FUNGI

Fungi (yeasts, moulds etc) are eukaryotic organisms, characterised by the absence of chlorophyll, the presence of a rigid cell wall in some stages of their life cycle, and their reproduction by means of spores. Their cell size ranges between 10-30 μm, containing organelles such as mitochondria, Golgi apparatus, lysosomes and endoplasmic reticulum, and linear DNA contained in a nuclear membrane. The cells are non-motile and heterotrophic. Their reproduction is complex (asexual and sexual).

There are two major morphological forms of fungi, small round yeasts and long filaments called hyphae. Yeasts are round, unicellular and multiply by budding or by fission. Filamentous fungi form hyphae; long tubes containing protoplasm which may have cross walls, called septa, which possess a central pore allowing the through flow of protoplasm; or may simply be multinucleate. A collection of hyphae is known as a mycelium, which may be vegetative, growing on a nutrient surface, or can extend upward as an aerial mycelium producing 'spores' (conidia) which spread very easily.

Dimorphic fungi exist in both forms. Many pathogenic fungi are dimorphic, usually with the yeast variety forming inside tissues and the filamentous (mould) form in the environment or surface.

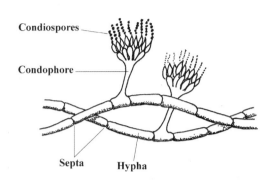

Condiospores

Condophore

Septa   Hypha

Structure of a filamentous mould

In terms of meat quality, fungi can survive on medium with a lower Aw than bacteria, and are less affected by pH. Different fungal groups produce varying physical appearances on meat, white 'whiskers' are attributable to *Mucor spp.*, green patches to *Penicillium spp.*, white spots to *Sporotrichum spp.*, and black spots to *Cladosporium spp.* They do, however, take longer to grow than bacteria, and meat spoilage is more likely to be attributable to the latter.

Various fungi produce chemicals during their growth such as antibiotics, and toxins known as mycotoxins. These secondary products of metabolism are not necessary for the growth of the fungi, but are felt to form a system to prevent competition for available space and nutrient from bacteria and other fungal species by inhibiting the growth of these other microorganisms. The antibiotics disrupt the growth of bacteria, the use of *Penicillium* spp. as an antibiotic is well known. Mycotoxins, when produced by fungi on foodstuffs such as grain kept in a humid environment can cause toxaemia in animals. The effects of which vary according to the level of toxin in the feedstuff, the duration of intake, and the age, sex and nutritional status of the host. Fungal toxins generally affect the liver.

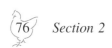

DISEASES OF POULTRY

AMYLOIDOSIS

Type	Miscellaneous
Aetiology	The deposition of an insoluble, starch like substance called amyloid in serous tissue.
Pathogenesis	When amyloid infiltrates tissue it becomes waxy and ceases to function. The deposition of amyloid is associated with chronic conditions such as tuberculosis, arthritis and environmental stressors.
Gross lesions	Ascites, sandy coloured, enlarged liver described as being par-boiled. Vegetative endocarditis, enlargement of the spleen with associated rupture.
Judgement	Offal unfit for human consumption. Assess carcase on its merits.
Other	The incidence increases with age.

ANATIPESTIFER

Synonyms	New Duck Disease. Infectious serositis.
Type	Bacterial
Aetiology	*Pasteurella anatipestifer.*
Pathogenesis	Occurs in ducks 2-7 weeks of age
Clinical signs	Ocular and nasal discharge, coughing and sneezing. Tremors.
Gross lesions	Lesions vary on how acute the infection is. Congestion of lungs and beak. Pink liver, splenomegaly. Vent pale green. Pericarditis, Perihepatitis, inspissated pus in abdominal airsacs. Caseous Salpingitis, sinusitis. Ocular and nasal discharge, fibrinous exudate over liver and in pericardium.
Judgement	Carcase and offal are unfit for human consumption.

AORTIC RUPTURE

Synonyms	Dissecting Aneurysm, Internal Haemorrhage.
Type	Miscellaneous
Aetiology	Various factors including genetic susceptibility. Mainly occurs in rapid growing male turkeys. Copper deficiency has been linked to this condition.
Pathogenesis	Fat deposition in the walls of the blood vessels, especially the aorta lead to localised weakening and rupture
Clinical signs	Birds are found dead with paleness of the heads.
Gross lesions	Massive internal bleeding due to rupture of a blood vessel.

This normally occurs in the aorta in the region of the testes. The carcase is anaemic.

Judgement | Carcase and offal are unfit for human consumption.

ASPERGILLOSIS

Synonyms	Brooder pneumonia, mycotic pneumonia, pneumomycosis
Type	Fungal
Aetiology	Fungal infection. **Aspergillus flavus** and **A. fumigatus**
Pathogenesis	Inhalation of spores. **Zoonotic**. Farmer's Lung
Clinical signs	Loss of appetite, gasping, increased respiratory rate, increased thirst, emaciation.
Gross lesions	Greyish-white caseous nodules in lungs and thickened air sac membranes.
	Greenish moulds in airsacs in chronic form as the conidiophores develop.
Judgement	Total rejection if associated with emaciation or septicaemia. Carcase meat may be salvaged if localised, reject affected parts.
Differential diagnosis	Pulmonary Granulomas associated with *M.gallisepticum* infection, tuberculosis, salmonellosis, and coryza.

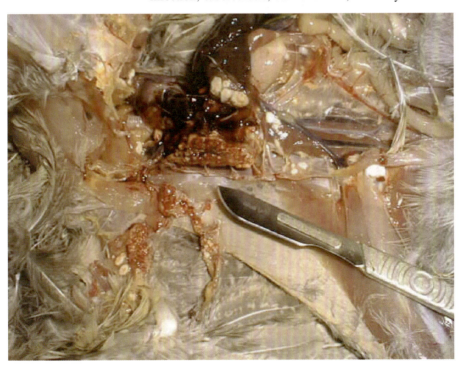

Aspergillosis lesions

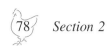

AVIAN CHLAMYDIOSIS

Synonyms	Ornithosis, Psitticosis.
Aetiology	*Chlamydia psittaci* closely related to Rickettsiae.
Pathogenesis	Inhalation or ingestion of faecal dust containing organism. Pigeons suspected as transport host.
Clinical signs	Chickens: Unobserved or mild respiratory infection.
	Turkeys: Nasal discharge, respiratory distress, green/yellow diarrhoea, loss of weight.
	Ducks: Anorexia, emaciation and watery diarrhoea.
Gross lesions	Chickens: Fibrinous pericarditis and enlarged liver.
	Turkeys: Wasting, vascular congestion, fibrinous inflammation of pericardium, air sacs and lungs, congestion of the lungs and enlarged, congested spleen.
	Ducks: Lacrimation, conjunctivitis, rhinitis and sinusitis, wasting of breast muscle, pericarditis, enlarged liver and spleen, Perihepatitis and peritonitis.
Judgement	Carcase and offal are unfit for human consumption.
Other information	**Zoonotic**. Known as psittacosis in humans and psittacine birds. Humans infected by inhalation or inoculation of faecal dust containing organism.

AVIAN INFLUENZA

Synonyms	Fowl Plague
Type	Viral
Aetiology	**Orthomixovirus** Types A, B or C
Clinical signs	Decreased activity, loss of appetite, emaciation, reduced egg production. Watery diarrhoea, cyanosis of comb, oedema of the wattle.
	Respiratory signs vary including sneezing, coughing, sinusitis and lacrimation.
	Eggs are quite often found without shells.
	Occasionally a diffuse haemorrhage may be found between the hocks and the feet.
Gross lesions	Highly Virulent – Congestion and haemorrhage on skin, liver, spleen, heart, kidneys and lungs, petechial haemorrhages in abdominal fat.
	Low Virulent – Lesions of the respiratory tract, sinusitis with mucopurulent to caseous exudate.
Judgement	Carcase and offal unfit for human consumption.
Differential diagnosis	Newcastle Disease, Fowl Cholera, Chlamydiosis, Mycoplasmosis.
Other	**Notifiable** in UK.

AVIAN SALMONELLOSIS

Synonyms	Paratyphoid.Used to describe Salmonella spp infections other than *S.gallinarum* and *S.pullorum*.
Type	Bacterial
Aetiology	10-12 species of Salmonella, commonest being **Salmonella typhimurium** in birds under one month of age.
Pathogenesis	Motile bacteria contaminate the egg in the oviduct, or during passage through the cloaca. Mechanical spread and also feedstuff containing animal protein has been incriminated.
Clinical signs	Drooping wings, shivering and huddling near heat source, muscular trembling.
Gross lesions	Enteritis associated with dehydration. Congested livers sometimes with haemorrhagic streaks. Unabsorbed yolk material. Omphalitis. Nodular lesions on pancreas, button-like lesions on intestines.
Judgement	Carcase and offal unfit for human consumption.

AVIAN MYCOPLASMOSIS

Synonyms	Chronic Respiratory Disease (CRD) Infectious Sinusitis
Aetiology	**Mycoplasma gallisepticum** (MG) (Chicken and Turkey), **Mycoplasma meleagridis** (MM) (turkey)
Pathogenesis	Often exacerbated by secondary infection by *E.coli*. Transmission by infected chickens, vertical transmission from hatchery. In acute form, infection is found in most tissues, however the epithelial cells of the respiratory system are most prone. MM is primarily egg transmitted through genital contact of contaminated sperm from the male to female.
Clinical signs	In cases uncomplicated by secondary infections there may be no clinical signs. Affected birds may show varying signs of respiratory distress including sneezing, rales and coughing. Swelling of the infra-orbital sinuses is common in turkeys, the inflammation almost closing the eyes. Ocular discharge is common in both species.In more complicated cases, infection can localize in synovial joints causing swelling.
Gross lesions	**MG** – Varying degrees of sinusitis, tracheitis and airsacculitis. Complication with *E.coli* gives rise to purulent, fibrinous pericarditis, perihepatitis and severe airsacculitis. **MM** – Airsacculitis. Has also been implicated in bone deformity (Perosis) including crooked necks.
Judgement	Reject affected parts. If emaciated or associated with systemic secondary infection then carcase and offal are unfit for human consumption.

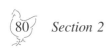

AVIAN TUBERCULOSIS

Synonyms	Avian T.B.
Type	Bacterial
Aetiology	***Mycobacterium avium***.
Pathogenesis	The disease begins with a primary focus; drainage from this leads to formation of lesions in adjacent lymphoid tissue and organs. This initial lesion causes the formation of tumour-like masses (tubercles) by stimulating the body's immune response. This formation is due to the covering of the infected area with dense, fibrous tissue, the subsequent tubercle formation normally prevents further spread of the infection. As the tubercle grows the centre, deprived of nutrients, dies (necrosis) and solidifies due to mineralisation. If bacteria escape from this area they travel via the blood and lymph stream and lodge in other areas of the body causing further tubercles to be formed.
Clinical signs	Dull, ruffled feather, pale skin and progressive emaciation.
Gross lesions	Greyish-white granulomatous nodular lesions of varying size in liver, spleen (which can become irregular in shape), intestinal serosa and in advanced cases in the bone marrow.
Judgement	Total Rejection
Differential diagnosis	Salmonellosis, fowl cholera, colibacillosis, Aspergillosis, chlamydiosis, typhoid and paratyphoid.
Other information	Tuberculous lesions are easily enucleated from surrounding tissue. Nodules in the intestinal serosa pass through the intestinal wall and discharge bacilli through ulcers into the intestines, from where they are passed out with the faeces.

BOTULISM

Synonyms	Limberneck, Western Duck Sickness.
Type	Bacterial
Aetiology	Exotoxins of ***Clostridium botulinum*** type A, C and E most common. *Cl.botulinum* is an anaerobic spore forming bacteria normally present in the soil.
Pathogenesis	*Cl.botulinum* types C and D are commensal organisms of the gastrointestinal tract of poultry. After ingestion of the toxin the clinical signs develop within 2-3 hours. This intoxication is through contaminated feed, decomposing carcases and beetles, maggots etc containing contaminant.
Clinical signs	Lack of coordination, weakness, diarrhoea. Flaccid paralysis of the neck and wings and/or legs.
Gross lesions	Intestines may be empty. Foul smelling contents in crop occasionally containing maggots may be found in cases of intoxication through spoilage of foodstuffs. Death may occur

without lesions developing through paralysis of the respiratory system.

Judgement | Carcase and offal are unfit for human consumption.

BREAST BLISTER

Synonyms	Sternal bursitis.
Type	Miscellaneous
Pathogenesis	Exudate produced forms blisters over the sternum when it is constantly bruised. This can occur through pressure on the sternum in cases of leg weakness or through jumping down from perches. Tends to occur in older, heavier birds especially turkeys.
Clinical signs	Normally the area above the bursa is partially denuded of feathers.
Gross lesions	Subcutaneous fluid forming a blister over the sternum.
Judgement	Trim affected parts and reject. If there is secondary infection of the blister (normally by *Staphylococcus aureus*) and septicaemia is evident then reject the entire carcase and associated offal as unfit for human consumption

CAGE LAYER FATIGUE

Synonyms	Cage layer paralysis.
Type	Nutritional
Aetiology	Demineralization of the skeletal structure.
Pathogenesis	Osteoporosis is a normal part of the egg-laying cycle. Calcium and phosphorous are removed from the bones of the laying fowl to provide the constituents of the eggshell. In cases of high production, combined with a lack of movement as can occur in battery systems, this depletion can be enhanced to the stage where it can become pathological in nature.
Clinical signs	Hens are found on their sides, normally with their legs extended and illustrate signs of paralysis. Death can follow rapidly. Bones are fractured easily; routine handling of the birds can produce fractures.
Gross lesions	Paralysis stems from fracture of the vertebrae producing compression of the spinal cord. Bone deformities are common, especially in the ribs and sternum. All the bones are thin and extremely fragile, fractures occur easily when the carcase is lifted.
Judgement	Carcases and offal are unfit for human consumption. The dangers of bone shards is too high to allow processing or consumption

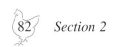

CANDIDIASIS

Synonyms	Thrush, Moniliasis, Sour Crop, Crop Mycosis
Type	Fungal
Aetiology	Yeast, ***Candida albicans***.
Pathogenesis	It has been suggested that the fungus in the crop may utilise or prevent the absorption of B vitamins.
Clinical signs	Depression and emaciation.
Gross lesions	Crop – thickened mucosa with raised, circular ulcer formation (Turkish towel effect). Occasionally haemorrhagic spots, necrotic foci and pseudomembranes.
Judgement	If associated with emaciation, the carcase and offal are unfit for human consumption.

CHICKEN ANAEMIA VIRUS

Synonyms	CAA (Chicken Anaemia Agent), Infectious Anaemia
Type	Viral
Aetiology	**Circovirus**
Pathogenesis	Depletion of lymphoid tissue, leading to atrophy and consequent immunosupression.
Clinical signs	Depression, paleness and weight loss.
Gross lesions	Anaemia, defective development of bone marrow (aplasia), bone marrow becoming fatty and yellowish. Enlarged, mottled livers, gangrenous dermatitis, atrophy of the thymus, spleen and bursa. Frequently the blood is watery, and haemorrhages can be observed in the proventriculus, and in subcutaneous and musculature systems.
Judgement	Carcase and offal unfit for human consumption.
Other information	Produces immunosupression, leading to complication with secondary infections.

CURLED TOE PARALYSIS

Type	Nutritional
Aetiology	Riboflavin deficiency
Pathogenesis	Affects birds up to 3 weeks of age.
Clinical signs	In-curling of toes, retarded growth, and emaciation. Weight supported on hocks.
Gross lesions	Sciatic nerve usually inflamed, up to 4-5 times normal diameter and yellowish appearance.
Judgement	Trim and reject affected parts. If emaciated, reject carcase and offal as unfit for human consumption.

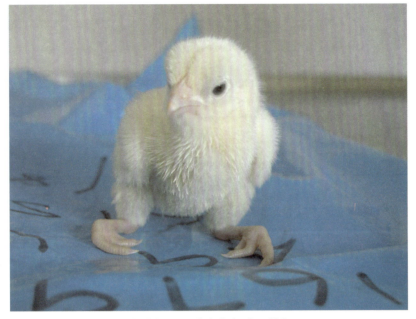

Curled toe paralysis in broiler chick

DUCK VIRUS ENTERITIS

Synonyms	Duck Plague.
Type	Viral
Aetiology	**Herpes virus**
Pathogenesis	Acute, contagious viral disease of ducks, geese and swans. Transmission is between infected birds and from the environment especially when birds have access to swimming water contaminated by free flying waterfowl. The incubation period is 3-7 days.
Clinical signs	Weakness, thirst, watery greenish-yellow diarrhoea, and soiled vents. Sticky ocular discharge, ruffled feathers, inability to stand, shows tremors, drooping, outstretched wings. Heads held down. Young ducks frequently have blood-soiled vents.
Gross lesions	Vascular changes lead to petechial haemorrhages and free blood in the body cavity. Crusty, diphtheric patches form in cloaca and oesophagus. Characteristic lesions include marked enteritis with necrosis of lymphoid tissue in Peyer's patches leading to macroscopic annular bands in the intestines. The liver may have focal necrosis.
Judgement	Total rejection of carcase and offal.

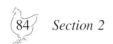

DUCK VIRUS HEPATITIS

Synonyms	DVH.
Type	Viral
Aetiology	**Picornavirus**
Pathogenesis	Affects ducklings between 2 days and 3 weeks of age, the clinical signs not seen in birds over 7 weeks old. Nearly all deaths occur within one week of infection.
	The virus infects orally, and can remain viable in infected faeces. Transmission is via mechanical carriers (wild birds) and wild duck (infected carriers.)
Clinical signs	Birds often in good condition will fall over sideways and struggle with spasmodic paddling movements and die within a few minutes. A characteristic sign of DVH death is the head stretched upwards and backwards, a condition known as opisthotonus.
Gross lesions	The liver is slightly enlarged, pale red and covered with haemorrhagic foci ranging from petechiae to 1cm in diameter. The spleen can be slightly enlarged and darker. The kidneys are normally enlarged with clearly visible surface blood vessel.
Judgement	Carcase and offal are unfit for human consumption.

EGG PERITONITIS

Synonyms	Yolk Peritonitis.
Type	Bacterial
Aetiology	*E.coli* **infection** of yolk in abdominal cavity.
Pathogenesis	Yolk freed into abdominal cavity due to ovarian regression, ovarian rupture and rising infection through oviduct, Salpingitis.
Clinical signs	Death, septicaemia, regression of laying.
Gross lesions	Yolk with cooked appearance amongst abdominal viscera. Peritonitis associated with foul smelling fluid.
Judgement	Carcase and offal unfit for human consumption.

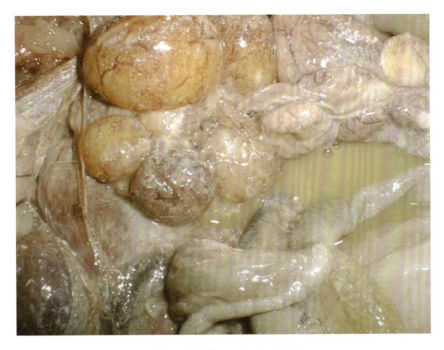

Egg peritonitis – note glary fluid

ERYSIPELAS

Synonyms	Leatherhead
Type	Bacterial
Aetiology	***Erysipelothrix rhusiopathiae***.
Pathogenesis	An acute septicaemia.
Clinical signs	Cyanosis of head due to vascular thrombosis, diarrhoea, pyrexia.
Gross lesions	Generalised septicaemia. Haemorrhages in muscle, subcutaneous fat and heart. Enlargement and congestion of liver and spleen. Catarrhal enteritis, endocarditis, fibrinopurulent exudate in joints.
Judgement	Carcase and offal unfit for human consumption.

EXUDATIVE DIATHESIS

Type	Nutritional
Aetiology	**Vitamin E deficiency** associated with selenium.
Pathogenesis	Increased vascular permeability allowing haemorrhage and plasma leakage.
Gross lesions	Accumulation of bloody fluid under the skin, especially over the area of the breast and under the wings. Hydropericardium and muscular oedema can also be present
Judgement	Carcase and offal are unfit for human consumption.

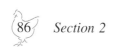

FAVUS

Synonyms	White Comb
Type	Fungal
Aetiology	Fungus ***Trichophyton meganinii***
Clinical signs	Greyish-white lesions cup-like spots on comb, coalescing to form a greyish-white crust over the face and wattles. In chronic cases the infection spreads to the head and neck, where the feathers fall out leaving a scaly, thickened area. This condition can lead to emaciation.
Judgement	Reject affected parts. If emaciated reject carcase and offal.

FEMORAL HEAD NECROSIS

Type	Miscellaneous
Aetiology	Inflammation of the cartilage (chondritis) and inflammation of the bone tissue (osteomyelitis) of the femur due to bacterial infection.
Pathogenesis	Degeneration and necrosis of the femur head associated with septicaemia, tenosynovitis, dehydration or emaciation.
Clinical signs	Lameness, signs of condition that produced FMH, i.e. septicaemia etc.
Gross lesions	The head of the femur is brittle and porous; the cartilage plate can be removed.
Judgement	If localised reject affected part. If produced as condition of systemic infection, or carcase is emaciated, reject carcase and offal as unfit for human consumption.

FOWL POX

Synonyms	Contagious epithelioma, Avian diphtheria.
Type	Viral
Aetiology	**Poxvirus**.
Pathogenesis	Spread by direct contact and mechanical vectors (e.g. biting insects).Two forms, wet and dry pox.
Clinical signs	Dry pox – Cutaneous form. Starts as small white bumps on comb, face and wattles. These grow rapidly turning yellow then brown, becoming scabby in 2-4 weeks. Egg production lowers.
	Wet form, breathing laboured, rapid weight loss.
Gross lesions	Wet form – Diphtheric form. Mucous membranes of mouth, throat and trachea become ulcerated with yellowish false membrane. These ulcers can coalesce to form complete false membrane that is difficult to remove and leaves raw, bleeding areas.

Judgement	Total rejection if generalised or associated with emaciation.
Other information	The dry, cutaneous form is often infected by secondary bacterial invasion.

FOWL TYPHOID

Type	Bacterial
Aetiology	***Salmonella gallinarum***.
Pathogenesis	Egg transmission, although mechanical transmission is also considered a possibility.
	Usually affects birds over 12 weeks of age.
	The causal organism can survive for 6 months in the environment under optimal conditions.
Clinical signs	Anorexia, diarrhoea
Gross lesions	Enlarged greenish-bronze coloured liver. Splenomegaly (may be mottled)
	Slimy enteritis of anterior intestines (white plaques in intestines of turkeys)
	Pale carcase.
	Petechial haemorrhages in muscles and fat, especially those areas adjacent to the internal organs.
Judgement	Carcase and offal are unfit for human consumption.

GANGRENOUS DERMATITIS

Synonyms	Necrotic Dermatitis, Gangrenous cellulitis, Avian Malignant Oedema.
Type	Bacterial
Aetiology	***Clostridium septicum***
Pathogenesis	Localised wounds in the skin lead to bacterial invasion. Several Clostridial spp of bacteria are associated with this condition with *Cl.septicum* being most prevalent. Certain disease complexes such as those leading to anaemia appear to reduce immunity to gangrenous dermatitis.
Clinical signs	Skin of legs and abdomen most affected.
Gross lesions	Skin necrosis, subcutaneous fluid, muscles have cooked appearance and hemorrhaging.
	Gas may also be produced under the skin and in the muscle tissue, producing a dry, crackling sound (crepitation) when the affected tissue is pressed.
Judgement	Carcase and offal are unfit for human consumption.

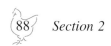

GOOSE VIRAL HEPATITIS

Synonyms	GVH. Derszy's Disease
Type	Viral
Aetiology	**Goose parvovirus type 1**
Pathogenesis	Acute disease of goslings and certain breeds of duckling under 4 weeks of age.
	Egg transmitted as well as direct contact.
Clinical signs	Conjunctivitis, nasal discharge, excessive thirst (polydipsia), huddling and death. Any feather loss is accompanied by reddened skin.
	In Muscovy ducks up to 3 months old sudden complete flock moulting has been recorded, followed by runting and stunting.
Gross lesions	Hepatitis and myocarditis associated with hydropericardium and ascites.
Judgement	Carcase and offal are unfit for human consumption.

GOUT

Type	Miscellaneous
Aetiology	Abnormal deposit of uric acid within joints or on viscera.
Pathogenesis	Two forms, visceral gout and articular gout. Articular gout is the less common form associated with high protein diets, affects individual birds possibly due to a genetic defect in the metabolism of uric acid. Visceral gout can affect individual birds or the flock, due to various factors such as water deprivation, kidney disease, Infectious bronchitis, avian monocytosis, obstruction of the ureters and Vitamin A deficiency.
Clinical signs	**Articular** – Slight lameness, possible emaciation. **Visceral** - Dehydration and uraemia.
Gross lesions	**Articular** – Semi-solid, white pasty material around joints, especially those of the feet and lower legs. **Visceral** – White, chalky deposits on serosal surfaces of internal organs, especially the liver, spleen and epicardium.
Judgement	**Articular gout** – Reject affected parts unless emaciated then entire carcase and offal unfit for human consumption. **Visceral gout** – Carcase and offal unfit for human consumption.
Other information	Urates are water-soluble.

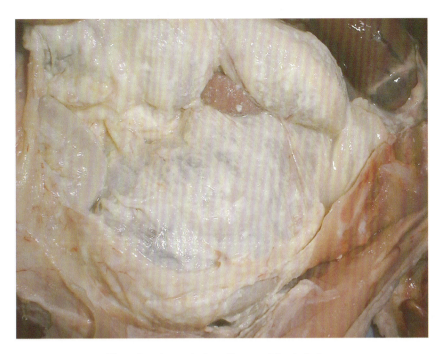

Visceral gout – urate deposition on abdominal viscera

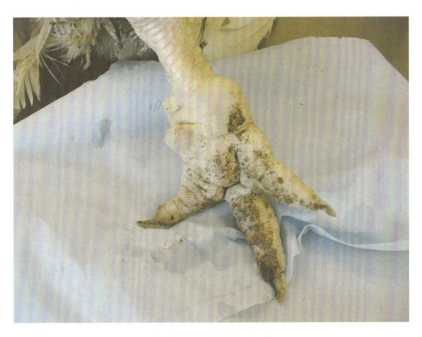

Articular gout affecting the foot

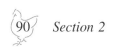

HAEMORRHAGIC ENTERITIS OF TURKEYS

Type	Viral
Aetiology	**Adenovirus**
Pathogenesis	Infection is gained via faecal-oral route; virion can remain infective for long periods in infected litter. Primary viral replication occurs in the spleen. Infection reduces immunity to secondary bacterial infections such as those caused by *E.coli*.
Clinical signs	Bloody droppings. Mortality can be up to 60%
Gross lesions	Enlarged, mottled spleen followed by atrophy and paleness. Blood in intestines (normally duodenum/jejunum) due to death and rupture of epithelial villi tips
Judgement	Reject affected parts, assess carcase on merits.

ICTERUS

Synonyms	Jaundice
Type	Miscellaneous
Aetiology	Deposition of bile pigments in the body tissues due to increased levels of bilirubin in the blood (hyperbilirubinaemia.)
Pathogenesis	Jaundice in birds occurs less frequently in avian species than in mammals due to the fact that bilirubin only forms approximately 6% of bile in birds. The increased levels of bilirubin in the blood are normally due to disturbances in the function of the liver system, associated with a failure to remove bile pigments from the intestine by means of the portal vein.
Clinical signs	Clinical signs vary with the nature of the cause of the hepatic disturbance. Unfeathered areas of skin appear yellow; in severe cases the eyes are coloured as too are the mucous membranes of the mouth.
Gross lesions	Tissues and organs of the body will be pigmented yellow; the liver is normally enlarged and yellow tinged.
Judgement	Carcase and offal are unfit for human consumption

IMPACTION OF THE OVIDUCT

Synonyms	Egg Impaction, Egg Bound
Type	Miscellaneous
Aetiology	Accumulation of egg yolk material, solid egg white and broken shell within the oviduct.
Pathogenesis	Can be due to cloacal infection, Salpingitis or vent pecking (a vice of laying fowl)
Gross lesions	Distended oviduct containing partly formed, misshapen eggs and caseous material.
Judgement	Reject affected parts if no secondary bacterial infection or septicaemia.

INCLUSION BODY HEPATITIS

Synonyms	Haemorrhagic Anaemia Syndrome
Type	Viral
Aetiology	**Adenovirus**
Pathogenesis	Thought to be vertically transmitted from parent flock, either in eggs or due to reduced parental antibody in the chicks. Horizontal transmission via bird-to-bird contact and equipment is thought to be the most likely course of the disease in the field.
Clinical signs	Initially IBH leads to deaths in apparently healthy birds. As the disease develops in the flock weakness, prostration, anaemia and jaundice of unfeathered skin are characteristic. Birds illustrating clinical lesions of IBH usually die within hours.
Gross lesions	Liver – pale and enlarged and mottled with haemorrhagic areas. Kidneys – Swelling and discolouration, often accompanied by uric acid crystals in the ureters. The spleen is generally enlarged and mottled. The bursa suffers atrophy and haemorrhages can be seen in muscles. In the anaemic form the bone marrow becomes pale.
Judgement	Carcase and offal are unfit for human consumption.

INFECTIOUS BRONCHITIS

Type	Viral
Aetiology	**Corona virus**
Pathogenesis	Incredibly contagious. Only affects chicken. Transmission by direct contact and airborne spread. Enters through trachea and lungs, where it replicates and enters bloodstream. Further replication occurs in other organs especially the oviduct. Damage to the kidneys can result in uraemia. Mortality is due to renal failure or to secondary infection.
Clinical signs	Respiratory – Normal characteristic signs of respiratory disease, including sneezing, gasping, rattling noises, facial swelling, tear production and watery nasal discharge. Reproductive – Egg production drops, egg quality deteriorates (shells thin, absent, smaller, yolks malformed, albumen watery).
Gross lesions	Respiratory – Airsacs cloudy, lungs congested, mucoid exudate in trachea. Reproductive – Atrophy of the oviduct, misshapen. Uraemic – Kidneys swollen and pale, ureters can be swollen and filled with uric acid crystals. Visceral gout can be produced.
Judgement	Unfit for human consumption if there is secondary involvement of the airsacs or visceral gout.

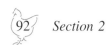

INFECTIOUS BURSAL DISEASE

Synonyms	Gumboro disease, Infectious Bursitis
Type	Viral
Aetiology	**Birna virus**
Pathogenesis	The virus primarily affects lymphoid tissue producing a progressive necrosis in the follicles of the bursa of Fabricius, destroying the lymphoid tissue and hence all the B-lymphocytes. T- cells, derived from the thymus appear unaffected. Unlike the bursa, the spleen, thymus and other lymphoid tissue is only affected in areas that B-cells normally congregate (for example the germinal follicles of the spleen) and the effects in these areas is reversible. The main effect of infection with the IBD virus is the destruction of B-lymphocytes and hence the reduction in humoral immunity; this immunosupression reduces vaccine response and the ability to defend against other diseases. The cell-mediated immunity provided by the T-cells remains unaltered.
Clinical signs	Whitish or watery diarrhoea, anorexia, depression and prostration. Occasionally vent pecking and trembling.
Gross lesions	Petechial haemorrhage in the muscles of the thigh and at junction of the proventriculus and gizzard may be seen. Inflammation of the bursa, which is severely enlarged, haemorrhagic and oedematous; by the fifth day of infection the size returns to normal, followed by atrophy of the organ which decreases to a third of the original size by the eighth day. There may be slight splenomegaly, with small grey foci on the surface.
Judgement	Carcase and offal are unfit for human consumption.

INFECTIOUS LARYNGOTRACHEITIS

Synonyms	ILT
Type	Viral
Aetiology	**Herpes virus** of the simplex group.
Pathogenesis	Turkeys and ducks appear resistant to the virus. Mainly affects chicken between 5-9months old. Three forms, subacute, acute and chronic. **Subacute form** – lesions appear within 2-3 days. Mortality 10-30%. **Acute form** – Sudden onset some days after infection. Mortality 50-70%. **Chronic form** – Months after initial infection. 1-3% mortality. Infection gained via respiratory tract or conjunctiva by contact with coughed up blood or mucous. The virus does not last long in the environment

Clinical signs	**Subacute** – Excess tear production (lacrimation), mild rattling in throat (rales), tracheitis and conjunctivitis.
	Acute –Head/neck extended during inhalation. Gasping, coughing, rales. Violent headshakes in attempt to remove obstruction from trachea, mouth sometimes bloodstained from tracheal exudate. Occasionally head parts become cyanotic.
	Chronic –Occasional coughing spasms and gasping when handled or excited. Nasal and ocular discharge.
Gross lesions	**Subacute** –haemorrhagic areas and yellowish diphtheric membrane in the larynx and upper third of respiratory tract, conjunctivitis.
	Acute –Mucous and yellow caseous exudate that sometimes forms a hollow cast in the trachea, haemorrhagic tracheitis. Death occurs by asphyxiation.
	Chronic –Necrotic and diphtheric patches in larynx, trachea and mouth.
Judgement	If emaciated, associated with secondary infection of the airsacs, the carcase and offal are unfit for human consumption.
Other information	The chronic form is easily confused with the diphtheric form of fowl pox.

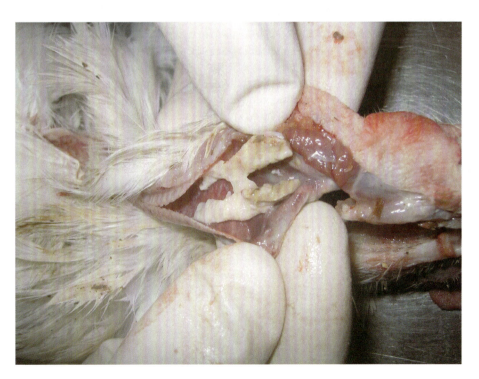

ILT – Caseous cast in trachea

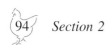

INFECTIOUS CORYZA

Type	Bacterial
Aetiology	*Haemophilus gallinarum*
Pathogenesis	Transmission by direct contact, airborne droplets and contamination of drinking water.
Clinical signs	Oedema and swelling around the eyes and wattles. Fluid exudate from the eyes can glue the eyelids together. Watery mucous from the nasal passages and swollen sinuses.
Gross lesions	Greyish, semi-fluid exudate in infraorbital sinuses. Secondary infection by other bacterial species can form purulent brownish/yellow exudate and extend infection into bronchitis and airsacculitis.
Judgement	Reject affected part. If carcase is emaciated, septicaemic or has purulent airsacculitis then carcase and offal are unfit for human consumption.

INFECTIOUS STUNTING

Synonyms	Infectious Stunting Syndrome (ISS), Malabsorption Syndrome. Infectious proventriculitis.
Type	Viral
Aetiology	**Reovirus**
Pathogenesis	Affects chickens 1-6 weeks of age. Lateral spread is associated with poor hygiene and increased stocking density. Viral agent survives in hens that may provide egg transmission but also may confer a certain amount of maternal immunity.
Clinical signs	Affected birds are thin with restricted growth. Faeces may contain undigested feed. Runts appear active.
Gross lesions	Varies from country to country, lesions produced form part of a syndrome. Inflammation of the proventriculus can occur; in some cases the organ becomes larger than the gizzard. Blockage of the pancreatic ducts due to inflammation is thought to be the cause of pancreatic atrophy and fibrosis. Arthritis may occur.
Judgement	Possible rejection on the grounds of contamination in machinery due to variation from flock norm and also before slaughter on welfare grounds.

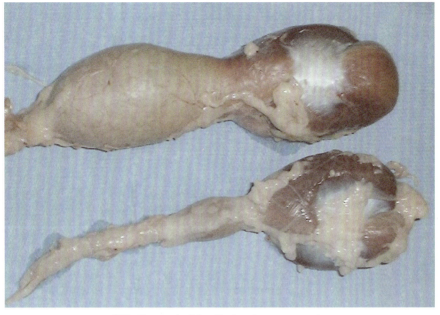

ISS - Proventriculitis affecting the upper sample

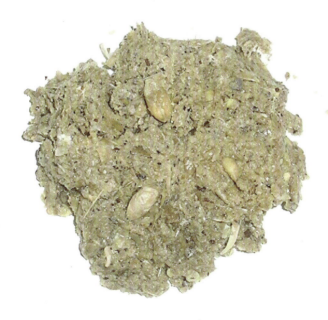

ISS – Malabsorbed material in droppings

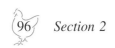

INFECTIOUS SYNOVITIS

Synonyms	Avian Mycoplasmosis, MS
Type	Bacterial
Aetiology	***Mycoplasma synoviae***
Pathogenesis	Egg transmission as with other avian mycoplasma. Bird to bird transmission also takes place.
Clinical signs	Lameness with swelling of joints, particularly those of the hocks and footpads. Rapid loss of condition, dehydration and diarrhoea.
Gross lesions	Inflamed joints and synovial membranes containing mucoid exudate. Can affect the wings as well as the legs. Inflammation of the sternal bursa can also be found to occur. Visceral lesions include greenish, enlarged livers, splenomegaly and airsacculitis.
Judgement	Depends on body condition and generalization of lesions. Ranges from rejection of affected joints to complete rejection if emaciation or systemic infection is present.

MARBLE SPLEEN DISEASE

Synonyms	Lung Oedema
Type	Viral
Aetiology	**Avian adenovirus**
Pathogenesis	An affection of pheasants causing necrosis of lymphoid cells in the spleen and hyperplasia of the white pulp producing a marbled effect.
Clinical signs	Depression is a clinical sign; however the first sign is, characteristically, death of the bird.
Gross lesions	The spleen is enlarged and mottled and lungs become oedematous and congested.
Judgement	Reject offal, assess carcase on merits.

MELANOSIS

Type	Miscellaneous
Pathogenesis	Melanin is a normal protein based pigment of the body, which colours the feathers, face, palate etc of birds. It can occur in abnormal amounts within the body, especially tissues such as the lungs, kidneys and spinal cord. Melanosis is congenital and the deposits are laid down in the foetus.
Gross lesions	The deposits are jet black, varying in size and shape and normally resembles ink splashes.
Judgement	Reject affected parts as unfit for human consumption.

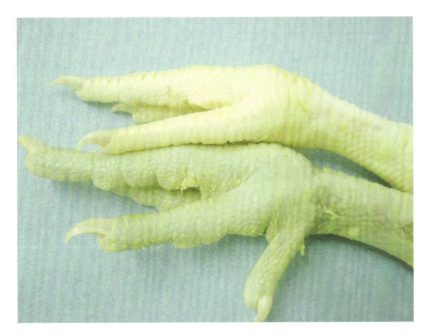

Broiler feet – the lower from a carcase affected with Melanosis

MYCOTOXICOSIS

Synonyms	Aflatoxicosis, Turkey X disease.
Type	Fungal
Aetiology	**Fungal toxin** poisoning. Aflatoxicosis due to the *Aspergillus flavus* mycotoxin.
Pathogenesis	Fungal mycotoxin produced on feedstuffs is ingested. Food left on the ground in close proximity to water feeders can promote fungal growth and possible toxin formation. The level of toxin ingested, combined with the period of consumption of the toxin determines the detrimental effects encountered.
Clinical signs	Lethargy, loss of appetite, death. Spasm of neck muscles, legs fully extended.
Gross lesions	Turkey – congestion and oedema of carcase, liver most affected. Chronic lesions include cirrhosis, the liver becoming yellowish-brown or mottled, hydropericardium, swollen kidneys. Ducks – Acute – liver and kidneys enlarged and pale. Chronic – cirrhosis, ascites and tumours in the liver.
Judgement	Carcase and offal are unfit for human consumption.

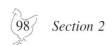

NECROTIC ENTERITIS

Synonyms	Cauliflower gut, Rot gut.
Type	Bacterial
Aetiology	***Clostridium perfringens***.
Pathogenesis	*Cl.perfringens* tends to be a secondary invader of the digestive tract. Predisposing factors for clostridial infection include coccidiosis, damage to the intestinal mucosa by toxins, variations in the rate of peristalsis due to changes in diet.
	Necrosis of the mucosa is thought to be due to clostridial toxins produced by the bacterial colonies.
	Necrotic enteritis tends to be associated with old, built up litter from which spores of *Cl.perfringens* are ingested.
Clinical signs	Affected birds can die within hours. Marked depression and occasional diarrhoea.
Gross lesions	Enlargement and congestion of the liver.
	The small intestines are ballooned and easily broken, contain foul smelling brownish contents and the mucosa is covered with a necrotic diphtheric membrane. Patches of this membrane can be described as vegetative, giving rise to the common name of cauliflower gut.
Judgement	Carcase and offal are unfit for human consumption.

NEWCASTLE DISEASE

Synonyms	Fowl pest. Avian pneumoencephalitis.
Type	Viral
Aetiology	Extremely virulent **paramyxovirus**. 5 Forms:
	Viscerotropic velogenic. (VVND)
	Neurotropic velogenic (NVND)
	Mesogenic
	Lentogenic respiratory
	Asymptomatic enteric
Pathogenesis	Highly contagious, all the birds in a flock can become infected within 3-4 days. Transmission via vectors such as free flying birds, fomites. Aerosol spread by infected birds also possible as faecal/oral.Recovered birds are not considered carriers and the virus remains viable in the environment for up to 30 days.
Clinical signs	Gasping, coughing, rattling in trachea, loss of appetite, huddling near heat sources.
	Nervous symptoms develop 1-2 days after respiratory including partial or complete paralysis of legs or wings. The head is held back between the shoulders or down between the legs (torticollis). Other features of the nervous form can include: walking backwards, circling and tumbling.

Gross lesions	VVND is most virulent, death normally occurring before the onset of symptoms. Those that can occur are severe haemorrhage and necrosis of the digestive tract especially the proventriculus and caecal tonsils
	Other forms include excess mucous in the trachea, bronchopneumonia and the cloudy appearance of airsacs.
Judgement	Carcase and offal are unfit for human consumption.
Other information	**Notifiable** in UK. Can increase incidence and be further complicated by secondary bacterial infections such as colibacillosis.

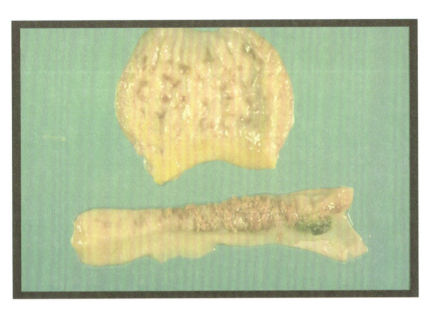

VVND – Haemorrhages in the proventriculus and caecal tonsils

OREGON DISEASE

Synonyms	Green muscle disease, deep pectoral myopathy.
Type	Miscellaneous
Aetiology	Ischaemic necrosis of the deep pectoral muscle *(M. supracoracoideus)*.
Pathogenesis	The covering (fascia) of the supracoracoideus muscle is inelastic and does not allow gross expansion of the muscle during intense exertion. This, coupled with the increased size of the pectoral muscle, can lead to occlusion of the blood supply to the supracoracoideus producing muscular necrosis.

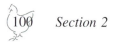

Clinical signs	Live birds show no apparent signs of discomfort or pain. Oregon disease in its early stages may be seen as a unilateral or bilateral swelling of the chest muscles and in its later stages as a 'dishing' of one or both muscles.
Gross lesions	In the early stages the muscle becomes swollen and reddish brown surrounded by excessive gelatinous fluid, eventually becoming atrophied, greenish and dry as necrosis develops.
Judgement	Affected muscle is rejected as unfit for human consumption.
Other information	Can be seen in turkeys by inserting a bright light source into the body cavity, necrotic breast muscle appears as a shadow. Can be unilateral or bilateral.

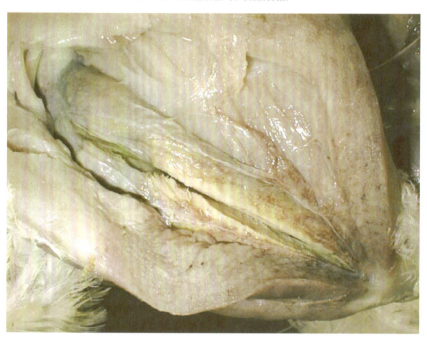

Deep pectoral myopathy – incision through pectoral muscle to supracoracoideus

PARACOLON INFECTION

Synonyms	Arizona infection, arizonosis (Mostly turkeys.)
Type	Bacterial
Aetiology	***Arizona hinshawi*** (formerly ***Salmonella arizoniae***)
Pathogenesis	Egg transmission though shells contaminated with faeces. Aerosol spread and direct contact with infected birds.
Clinical signs	Listlessness and trembling, faecal contamination of the vent area.

	Twisting of head and neck.
	Cloudiness and swelling of eye causing blindness.
	Affected birds seen huddling near a light source.
Gross lesions	Enlarged yellow liver. Congestion of duodenum. Inflammation of oviduct (Salpingitis) and peritoneum. Small focal lesions in lungs.
Judgement	Carcase and offal unfit for human consumption.

PASTEURELLOSIS

Synonyms	Fowl Cholera
Type	Bacterial
Aetiology	***Pasteurella multocida***.
Pathogenesis	Three forms, peracute (septicaemic), acute and chronic. Organism can survive for months in decaying carcases and moist soil, and is also common in wild and domestic animals such as rodents and carnivores.
Clinical signs	Peracute – sudden death.
	Acute – Listlessness, refusal to drink, loss of flesh, diarrhoea, cyanosis of head
	Chronic – Cyanosis, swelling of wattles and snood.
Gross lesions	Peracute – Petechial haemorrhages in heart, liver, proventriculus, gizzard and intestines. Liver streaked with light areas and greyish-white necrotic foci.
	Acute – Few or none.
	Chronic – Abscesses in wattles. In laying flocks, cheesy material (ruptured egg yolks) in body cavity with putrid smell. Swelling of tendon sheaths common.
Judgement	Carcase and offal are unfit for human consumption.

PEROSIS

Type	Nutritional
Aetiology	**Manganese deficiency**.
Pathogenesis	Deformity of the long bones
Clinical signs	Leg pulled sideways due to displacement of *gastrocnemius* tendon from its guiding condyles at the rear of an enlarged tibiotarsal joint
Judgement	If localised reject affected part. If associated with emaciation carcase and offal are unfit for human consumption.

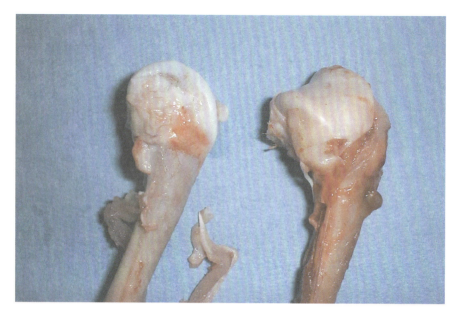

Perosis – deviation of the tibial chondial apparent in tibia on right

PSEUDOTUBERCULOSIS

Type	Bacterial
Aetiology	***Yersinia pseudotuberculosis***
Pathogenesis	Host to host, although rodents have been associated with spread. Infection through intestinal mucosa or breaks in the skin set up a bacteraemia.
Clinical signs	Birds can be found dead with no symptoms. Chronic cases show chronic diarrhoea, weakness, dehydration and emaciation.
Gross lesions	Acute – Enlargement of liver and spleen. Less acute – tubercle-like lesions, yellow/white necrotic foci in liver, spleen and lungs. Severe enteritis.
Judgement	Carcase and offal unfit for human consumption.

PULLORUM DISEASE

Type	Bacterial
Aetiology	***Salmonella pullorum***
Pathogenesis	Primarily egg transmitted. Further spread due to direct contact, carrier birds and infected premises. Routes of entry into body are the respiratory and digestive systems.
Clinical signs	Anorexia, diarrhoea, pasting of vents.
Gross lesions	Grey nodules ranging in size from pinhead to pea size in lungs, liver, heart, intestine, peritoneum, gizzard (under cutica gastrica) and spleen.
Judgement	Carcase and offal unfit for human consumption.

RICKETS

Type	Nutritional
Aetiology	**Vitamin D deficiency**.
Clinical signs	Poor growth rate, feather development poor, beak and claws become soft and pliable.
Gross lesions	Skeletal deformities especially in the legs and ribs (nodules on inner surface). Bones become soft and pliable.
Judgement	Carcase and offal unfit for human consumption.

SPONDYLOLISTHESIS

Synonyms	Kinky back
Type	Miscellaneous
Aetiology	This condition only affects broiler birds. The free thoracic vertebrae (T4) suffers a downward rotation, this may crush the spinal cord in the vertebral channel leading to paralysis of the lower limbs.
Pathogenesis	This condition appears hereditary, and occurs in broilers with high initial growth rates; reducing the initial growth rate by food intake reduction prevents this condition.
Clinical signs	The bird is unable to rise and is seen squatting on its hocks. When attempting to move a characteristic 'back peddling' of the wings is a common feature.
Gross lesions	Downward rotation of the T4 vertebra.
Judgement	Fit unless the carcase is emaciated.
Differential diagnosis	Clinical Signs – Marek's Disease, Osteomyelitis of the vertebral column.

SWOLLEN HEAD SYNDROME

Synonyms	Avian rhinotracheitis, 'swell head'
Type	Viral
Aetiology	Avian **Pneumovirus**
Pathogenesis	Contact spread. Nasal discharge, fomites such as contaminated water, contaminated equipment; contaminated feed trucks and load-out activities can contribute to the transmission of the virus, egg transmission is also a possibility.
Clinical signs	Periorbital swelling – subcutaneous oedma starting around the eyes that extends over the entire head, resting of head on back (opisthotonus)
Gross lesions	Incision of skin overlying lesion reveals yellowish fluid which may become seropurulent. Secondary infection may lead to airsacculitis.
Judgement	Reject affected parts. If associated with emaciation or secondary systemic bacterial infection reject entire carcase and offal.

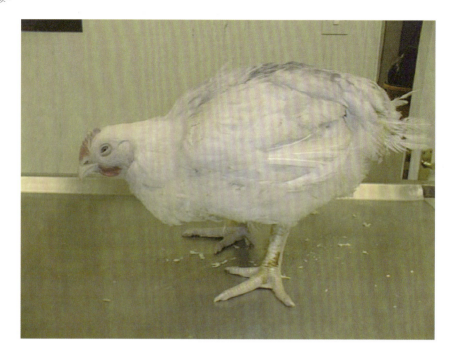

Periorbital oedema associated with Swollen Head Syndrome

TIBIAL DYSCHONDROPLASIA

Synonyms	Focal Osteodystrophy.
Type	Miscellaneous
Aetiology	Persistent mass of hypertrophic uncalcified cartilage in the proximal end of the tibiotarsal bone.
Pathogenesis	Particularly common in ducks. Due to a combination of dietary (acid/base balance) and genetic factors.
Clinical signs	Lameness. Bowing of tibiotarsus. If hypertrophy is severe can lead to pathogenic fracture of the bone due to lateral pressure.
Judgement	Reject affected parts unless carcase is emaciated.

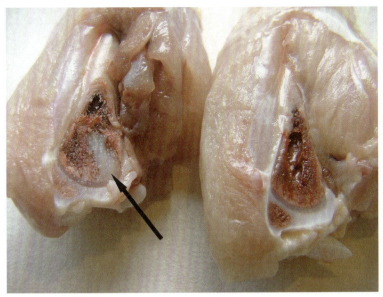

Tibial dyschondroplasia – persistant mass of cartilage in left hand sample (arrowed)

TRANSMISSIBLE ENTERITIS OF TURKEYS

Synonyms	Bluecomb
Type	Viral
Aetiology	**Coronavirus**
Pathogenesis	Acute or chronic disease. Transmission via infected birds or premises, viral agent survives in faeces. Acute form affects turkey poults around 3-4 weeks of age.
Clinical signs	Birds seek heat sources. Food and water consumption drops. Rapid weight loss. Diarrhoea Chronic – cyanosis of head, droppings containing mucous.
Gross lesions	Acute - Intestines distended, contents watery and foamy (gas.) Chronic – dehydration, multiple white chalky areas on pancreas, catarrhal enteritis. Petechial haemorrhages on viscera, excess urates.
Judgement	Acute - If emaciated reject carcase and offal. Chronic – Reject carcase and offal.

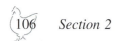

ULCERATIVE ENTERITIS

Synonyms	Quail disease.
Type	Bacterial
Aetiology	***Clostridium colinum***.
Pathogenesis	Oral infection, normally as secondary opportunistic invader after primary infection with diseases such as IBD or coccidiosis. Colonizes lower intestine. Liver lesions produced when organism passes through portal system.
Clinical signs	Acute infection leads to death of healthy, normal birds. Chronic infection, characteristic droppings streaked with white urate and surrounded with a watery ring. Birds become listless, huddled with neck retracted.
Gross lesions	Enteritis of the lower third of the small intestine, leading to button-like ulceration. Some ulcers may perforate intestines leading to peritonitis. Yellow, irregular focal necrosis is produced in the liver by invading organisms.
Judgement	Reject affected parts. If emaciation or septicaemia present, reject carcase and offal.

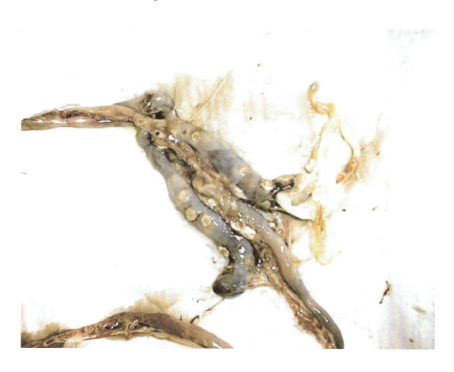

Ulcerative enteritis

VIRAL ARTHRITIS

Synonyms	Tenosynovitis, tendonitis
Type	Viral
Aetiology	**Reovirus**
Pathogenesis	Affects synovial membranes, tendon sheaths and the myocardium.
	Mainly affects chicken 4-16 weeks old. Infection occurs when young.
Clinical signs	Bilateral swelling of tendons. Stilted walk.
Gross lesions	Swelling and inflammation of the tendon sheaths above the hock and along the back of the shank (digital flexor and metatarsal extensor tendons). Rupture of the gastrocnemius tendon common. Acute lesion exudate in synovial spaces, leading to fibrosis in chronic cases. The liver, heart and spleen can become enlarged in chronic infections with necrotic foci developing.
Judgement	Reject affected parts. Reject carcase and offal if carcase is emaciated.

PARASITES

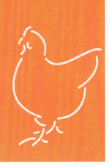

3

PARASITISM

Parasites can be defined as plants or animals that live on or within another living organism at whose expense it gains some advantage. The host/parasite association can be complicated.

Parasitic infections are not normally considered important in broiler production; the method of rearing tends to prevent access to the transport host of parasites, and the relatively short chick to slaughter lifespan (approximately 42 days) both contribute to the lack of economic loss and welfare problems due to parasites. However the modern trend toward free-range and organic poultry has once again given poultry access to 'uncontrolled environments' and contact with parasites of wild birds and insect vectors of poultry parasites.

The type of parasite encountered ranges from viruses (intracellular parasites) that can only reproduce in a living cell, to protozoa (single celled organisms) to intestinal worms and insects. Although they are parasitic, viruses are generally treated as a separate group, and we will only be considering parasites that are internal (endoparasites) and external (ectoparasites) that affect poultry.

Parasites may have a direct or indirect lifecycle. A direct lifecycle means that the parasite can only complete the life cycle by parasitising the host.

ENDOPARASITES

HOST / PARASITE RELATIONSHIP

The lifecycles of parasites vary, but endoparasites undergo a three-step association with the host animal. Firstly, the parasite must infect the host via the intestines or the skin. Secondly the individual parasite must be maintained within the host, this includes feeding, growth and migration within the host. Thirdly the species must be maintained, which means reproduction and the dispersal of the infective agents.

Each of these stages of association present different hurdles for the parasite.

INFECTION

Obviously the initial stage of parasitic development is gaining entry to the host animal. The parasite has to survive in some form in the atmosphere, whilst remaining available to enter the host. The lifecycle of most endoparasites includes a hibernation stage, for example as a cyst or egg, the infective agent, where the immature parasite lies dormant until suitable conditions trigger the release of the agent. The availability of the infective agent to host entry is achieved in various ways, some stages of a lifecycle

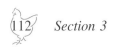

may include the infective agent existing in a secondary or intermediate host such as worms, beetles or ants that are ingested by the primary host. The single overriding factor in the availability of the infective agent to host entry is mathematical. Infection of the host is a matter of chance; the vast numbers of infective agents produced by the adult parasite increases the odds.

INDIVIDUAL MAINTENANCE

Once the agent has entered the hosts' body, by whatever means, it has to be able to migrate to its preferred site of habitation (predilection site), where it can mature. This can involve migration through body tissue or at the very least passage through the digestive system. Some parasites use the digestive process to activate the infective agent, others produce secretions to neutralise the effects of the gastric juices. The migration and settling of the immature parasite will also prompt the host animal's immune response to a foreign agent, this is overcome by some parasites by protective secretions.

PARASITE MAINTENANCE

On reaching the site where they mature, the parasite takes nutrients from the host to mature. A successful parasite can be considered as one that infects, lives, reproduces and infects other hosts without killing the primary host.

SPECIES MAINTENANCE

The role of any organism, from bacterium to human, is propagation of the species. Eggs and unsporulated oocysts are passed by mature poultry parasites in the faeces, and become infective agents.

The affects of parasites on the host can be dramatic and include physical blockage such as in the case of *Syngamus trachea* that can cause blockage of the trachea if in large numbers, and *Ascaridia galli,* an intestinal roundworm that can block the intestines as well as reducing nutrient intake. The presence of parasites within the body can also lower the host resistance to secondary infection by bacterial species and other parasites, as well as introducing infection themselves. *E.coli* is a common secondary invader of the body and the protozoan parasite *Histomonas meleagridis* (blackhead) is normally introduced to the body by the caecal worm *Heterakis gallinarum.*

PARASITE LIST

Common parasites of poultry include:

ENDOPARASITES

Protozoa / Rickettsiae

Histomonas meleagridis (Blackhead, infectious enterohepatitis)
Hexamita meleagridis
Eimeria spp. (Coccidiosis)

Helminths

Ascarids (Intestinal Worms)
Ascaridia galli
Ascaridia dissimilis (Turkeys)
Ascaridia columbae (Pigeons.)
Capillaria (Hair worms / Thread worms)
Capillaria contorta
Capillaria obsingata
Capillaria caudinflata
Heterakis gallinarum (Caecal worm)
Heterakis isolonche (Game birds)
Syngamus trachea (Gapeworm, Redworm)

ECTOPARASITES

Mites

Cnemidocoptes mutans (Scaly leg mite)
Cnemidocoptes gallinae (Depluming-itch mite)
Dermanyssus gallinae (Red Mite)
Laminosioptes cysticola (Tissue mite)
Ornithonyssus sylvarium (Northern Fowl Mite)

Fleas

Ceratophyllus gallinae (Poultry Flea)
Echidnophaga gallinacea ('Stick-tight' burrowing flea)

Lice

Menacanthus stramineus. (Body Lice)

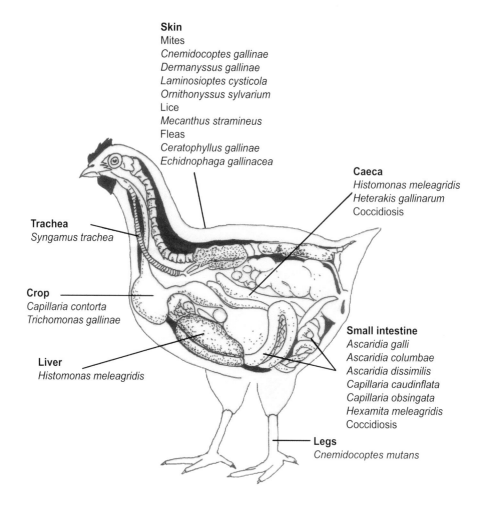

Skin
Mites
Cnemidocoptes gallinae
Dermanyssus gallinae
Laminosioptes cysticola
Ornithonyssus sylvarium
Lice
Mecanthus stramineus
Fleas
Ceratophyllus gallinae
Echidnophaga gallinacea

Caeca
Histomonas meleagridis
Heterakis gallinarum
Coccidiosis

Trachea
Syngamus trachea

Crop
Capillaria contorta
Trichomonas gallinae

Small intestine
Ascaridia galli
Ascaridia columbae
Ascaridia dissimilis
Capillaria caudinflata
Capillaria obsingata
Hexamita meleagridis
Coccidiosis

Liver
Histomonas meleagridis

Legs
Cnemidocoptes mutans

Common parasites of poultry

PROTOZOA

Protozoa are single-celled organisms that, unlike bacteria, possess a nucleus and other organelles that enable them to lead an independent existence. Protozoa are mobile organisms, using methods of propulsion such as flagella, cilia and undulating membranes. They feed by enveloping particles and digesting them, followed by the extrusion of waste material from the cell. In poultry the forms encoubnterd include *Eimeria species*, *Trichomonas species*, *Histomonas meleagridis* and *Hexamita meleagridis*.

COCCIDIOSIS

Coccidiosis is a disease condition caused by the actions of the coccidial protozoan parasite of the *Eimeria* genus.

In poultry *Eimeria spp.* are intercellular parasites of the cells that line the internal surface of the intestines (epithelial cells) and cause lesions by destroying the cells as part of their lifecycle. The severity of the disease is dependant on the number of infective agents ingested, but as an infected hen can pass several hundred million of these agents in faeces during the course of the disease, it is easy to see why coccidiosis can account for 5-10% of deaths in untreated poultry flocks. The use of preventative coccidiostats in broiler production is now standard practice, as the introduction of intensive husbandry methods has increased the risk of infection.

LIFECYCLE

There are three basic stages in the lifecycle of *Eimeria* species, **Sporulation** occurring outside the host, **infection / Shizogony**, and **Gametogony** and oocyst formation.

Sporulation – eggs, or oocysts (a resistant shell surrounding protoplasm and a nucleus) are passed in the faeces. Under optimum conditions, within 2-4 days the nucleus divides to produce four sporoblasts, each containing two sporozoites (the infective agent). The sporoblasts secrete a covering wall to form sporocysts. This make up, four sporocysts containing eight sporozoites are indicative of *Eimeria* species and is used as a diagnostic method.

Infection and Shizogony. (Asexual reproduction.) – When ingested by the host, either through eating vector organisms such as earthworms that have ingested oocyst, or by ingestion of oocysts during feeding, the sporocysts are liberated from the oocyst by the digestive processes of the host animal. The sporozoites are activated by the presence of bile and trypsin in the small intestine and leave the sporocyst, and are now known as trophozoites. The trophozoites enter epithelial cells in the intestine and forms schizonts, in which division of the trophozoites nucleus forms merozoites. When the shizont containing merozoites is mature, the shizont and host cell rupture, allowing the merozoites to enter other epithelial cells where the process is repeated.

Gametogony (Sexual reproduction.) – Eventually the merozoites enter a host cell and develop into either a male form (microgametocyte) containing microgametes (small, actively mobile, flagellated organisms, similar in function to sperm), or develop into the female form, the macrogametocyte, which are

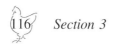

single celled and expand to fill the host cell. When the microgametocyte is mature, it ruptures, together with the host cell and releases the microgametes. One microgamete then enters the host cell containing the macrogametocyte, penetrates the latter, and fusion of the two nuclei takes place. A cyst wall then develops forming a zygote that is later released as an unsporulated oocyst in the faeces when the host cell ruptures

LIFECYCLE OF *EIMERIA SPP.*

Phase 1. Sporulation

Egg (oocyst) passed in faeces. Nucleus divides twice forming four sporoblasts. The content of each sporoblast divides into two, forming 8 sporozoites (the infective agent) per egg. The sporoblast secretes a wall to become a sporocyst. This stage occurs outside the host.

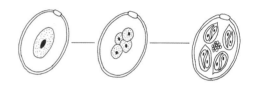

Phase 2. Infection and Shizogony

(Asexual reproduction)

When the sporulated oocyst is ingested the digestive processes of the host free the 4 sporocysts. Bile and trypsin in the intestines activate the 8 sporozoites, which leave the sporocysts. The sporozoites are now known as trophozoites enter host cells and develop into a shizont containing merozoites. When the schizont is mature it and the host cell rupture and the merozoites are released to invade neighbour cells. This process is repeated, the number of repetitions being species dependant.

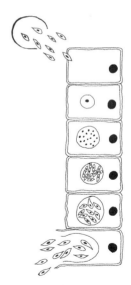

Phase 3. Gametogony

(Sexual Reproduction)

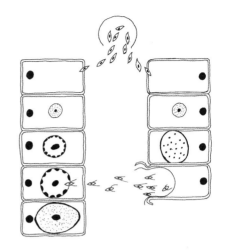

Eventually, merozoites entering host cells develop into either male microgametocytes or female macrogametocytes. The males undergo division to form mobile, flagellated microgametes within the microgametocyte. The female macrogametocyte enlarges to fill the host cell. When the male host cell ruptures, the microgametes are freed, when one enters the macrogametocyte the male and female nucleus combine. A cyst wall is formed creating an oocyst, which is passed in the faeces.

AFFECTS ON THE HOST

Eimeria species are host-specific, which is to say that a species that affects turkeys will not infect chickens and vice versa. Poultry, like other animals affected by species of Eimeria can develop certain immunity to infection from exposure previous infections, however this acquired immunity is again species specific, only relevant to the species of Eimeria encountered. The susceptibility to infection is also increased by the presence of other disease conditions that may lower the immune response, notably Infectious Bursal Disease (Gumboro) and Marek's disease.

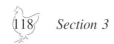

COCCIDIOSIS IN TURKEYS

Four main species of Eimeria are of importance in turkeys, these are shown below.

Species	Location of Infection	Lesions
E. meleagrimitis	Upper SI	Haemorrhagic lesions, casts, dilation of jejunum.
E. gallopavonis	Rectum	Ulceration and yellowish exudate.
E. meleagridis	Caeca	Creamy exudate, caseous core
E. adenoides	Lower SI and caeca	Petechial haemorrhages, mucoid exudate, caecal mucosa detaches producing caecal core.

COCCIDIOSIS IN CHICKENS

Six species of Eimeria are recognised in chicken, each with varying degrees of disease causing capability (pathogenicity), and affecting varying parts of the intestine. Differentiation between species is achieved by for example, location and type of lesion and the dimensions of the oocyst.

Species	Location of Infection	Lesions
Eimeria tenella	Caeca	Schizonts only develop in the mucosa. Haemorrhage, white spots, blood in faeces. Thickened mucosa, later core of clotted blood.
E. necatrix	Small intestine	Haemorrhage, thickening of intestinal wall. White spots on serosa. Distended intestines with blood inside. Can cause acute mortality in laying hens, weight loss and blood in faeces.
E. brunetti	Lower small intestine	Slight haemorrhage, coagulative necrosis, becoming fibrinous enteritis with a bloody mucoid exudate. Whitish blood streaked faeces.
E. acervulina	Upper small intestine	Watery exudate. White transverse bands of oocysts visible through intestinal wall. In heavy infestations the plaques coalesce and the intestinal walls thicken.
E. maxima	Mid small Intestine	Salmon pink exudate, thickened walls. Haemorrhage in heavy infections. Possesses large microgameto-cytes and oocysts.
E. mitis	Lower small intestine	No visible lesions.

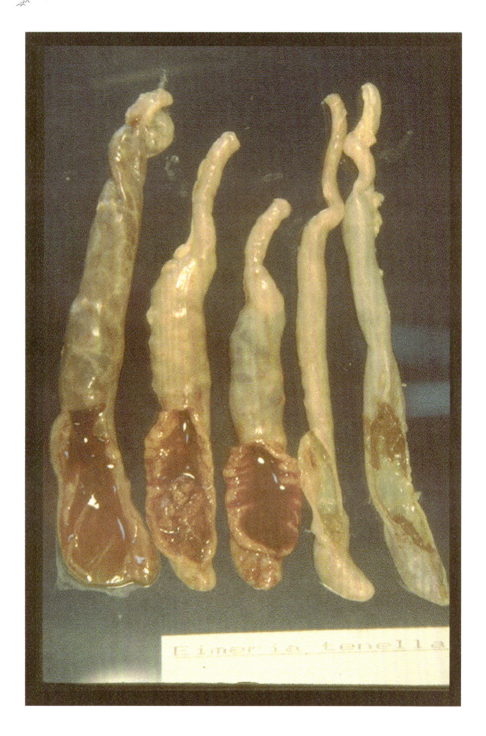

Lesions of *Eimeria tenella*

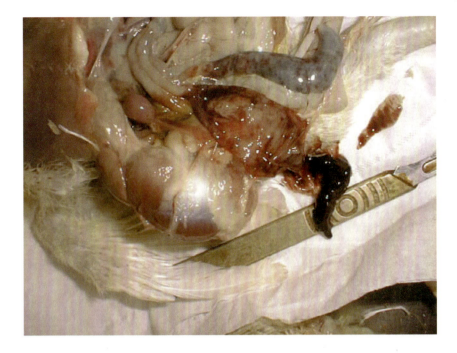

Caecal coccidiosis

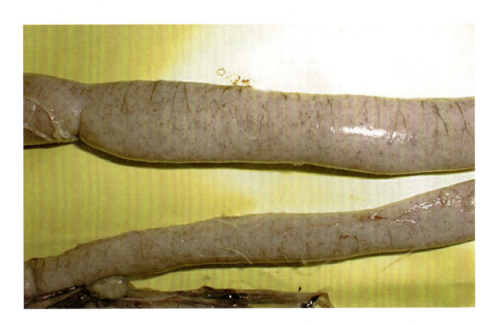

Eimeria necatrix lesions in serosa of intestines

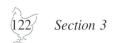

HISTOMONAS MELEAGRIDIS

Histomonas meleagridis is a protozoan parasite chiefly affecting young turkeys, which causes condition known as Blackhead, Histomoniais or infectious enterohepatitis. The lifecycle of *H.meleagridis* is unusual in that is uses the eggs (oocysts) of another parasite, the poultry caecal worm *Heterakis gallinarum*, as its mode of infection. It is thought that the adult *H.gallinarum* is infected, possibly by ingesting the histomonads whilst in the caeca, the flagellated larvae enter the ovaries of the worm and are passed inside the oocyst with the faeces of the fowl. The oocysts can then enter another host either direct from the ground, or by eating earthworms that have acted as a transport host by themselves ingesting infected oocysts of *H. gallinarum*, which either hatch in the worm producing viable larvae infected by histomonads, or remain as viable oocysts within the worm. When the oocysts of the caecal worm are ingested and hatch, the histomonads are released and enter the mucosa of the caeca, causing ulceration and necrosis. The histomonads can reach the liver via the portal blood circulation. There they colonise the liver substance and produce characteristic circular necrotic foci that increase in size as the parasites multiply in the periphery of the lesion.

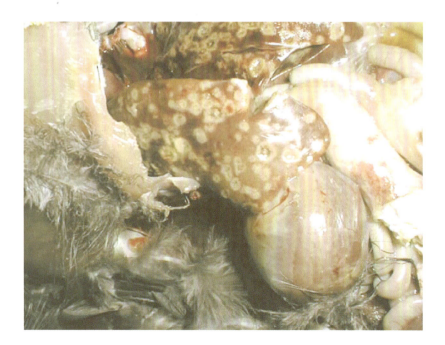

Histomoniasis lesions in a turkey liver

Turkey poults, eight days after infection become dull, with ruffled feathers and pass bright yellow faeces. If unchecked, or if the number of histomonads is sufficiently large, the birds can die within two weeks of infection.

Older turkeys tend to display a chronic wasting, normally followed by recovery and an acquired immunity to re-infection.

The term 'Blackhead" is applied due to the cyanosis of the head and wattles which was thought to be characteristic of this parasitic infection.

HEXAMITA MELEAGRIDIS

Hexamita meleagridis is a protozoal parasite of turkeys, pheasants, ducks and quail, which can cause acute, catarrhal enteritis. It is spindle shaped with 6 anterior and 2 posterior flagella by which it attaches to epithelial cells of intestines.

Transmission of these protozoa is direct via the faecal-oral route; game birds such as pigeons and pheasants have been implicated in the dissemination of infection throughout outdoor reared turkey flocks. Birds remain carriers after infection and can transmit *Hexamita meleagridis* to uninfected birds.

Clinical Signs include emaciation, rapid weight loss even though feed intake is normal, watery or foamy diarrhoea. Birds chirp excessively, have subnormal temperatures and huddle near heat sources. Birds then become depressed, stand with heads retracted with drooping wings.

Death can occur due to hypoglycaemia, a rapid reduction in the blood glucose levels causing convulsions and coma.

Gross Lesions found are enteritis with bulbous dilation of the small intestine, especially the duodenum and upper jejunum, which are filled with watery contents.

Reject offal as unfit for human consumption; unless the carcase is emaciated then reject carcase and offal

Hexamita columbae is found in the small intestines of pigeons and causes enteritis.

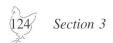

TRICHOMONAS GALLINARUM

Trichomonas gallinarum and *Trichomonas columbae* are protozoan parasites that cause conditions known by the synonyms of Canker and Frounce.

Although with the ability to affect all species, pigeons are most severely affected partly due to the parents feeding their young with 'crop milk', regurgitated desquamated lipid cells from the mucosa of the crop directly into the oropharynx of the young.

Soft tissue injury to the oropharynx appears to increase the invasive potential of the parasite which initially produces red ringed circumscribed lesions which can coalesce to form a yellowish material that can obstruct the oesophagus and trachea. The lesions may spread to the crop, proventriculus and respiratory passages.

Affected parts should be rejected as unfit for human consumption, if lesions lead to emaciation of the carcase the entire carcase and associated offal should be rejected as unfit.

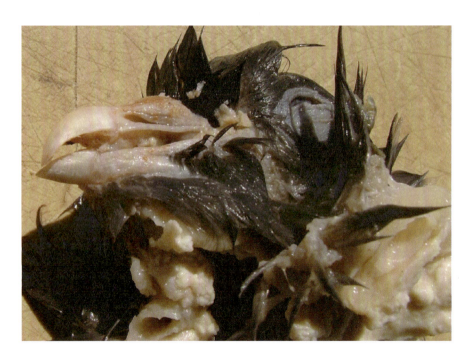

Yellow caseous lesions of 'Pigeon canker'. Sample fixed in formalin

HETERAKIS GALLINARUM

Heterakis gallinarum, also known as the caecal worm is possibly the commonest nematode worm parasite of poultry. They are whitish worms that have male and female forms that grow to 1.0-1.5 cm in length and inhabit the caeca. *Heterakis gallinarum* is, in itself, felt to be non-pathogenic to poultry, however, it is important as the carrier of the protozoan parasite *Histomonas meleagridis*, which produces infectious enterohepatitis or 'blackhead' in turkey poults.

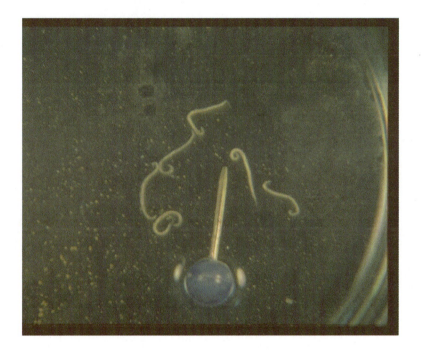

Heterakis gallinarum

Eggs are passed in the faeces of infected poultry and become infective within 2-3 weeks. Earthworms are recognised as important vectors of this parasite, either in their role of spreading the eggs further by ingesting and passing the eggs through their gut, or through the hatching of the eggs within the worm, where the larvae enter the tissues and remain viable until the worm itself is ingested by poultry.

Heterakis isolonche affects game birds, especially pheasants and differs from *H.gallinarum* in that the larvae burrow into the mucosa of the caeca and moult in nodules to form mature worms. Eggs are passed through openings in the nodules into the gut, where they are passed in faeces. Unlike *H.gallinarum*, *H.isolonche* produces pathogenic effects in the host including severe typhlitis with associated diarrhoea and progressive emaciation.

SYNGAMUS TRACHEA

Syngamus trachea is a helminth parasite affecting the upper respiratory tract, (the trachea, bronchi and bronchioles.) If present in large numbers, the inflammation produced can cause the condition known as 'gapes' where respiratory distress brought about by the physical blockage of the trachea leads to laboured breathing, outstretched necks and open mouths.

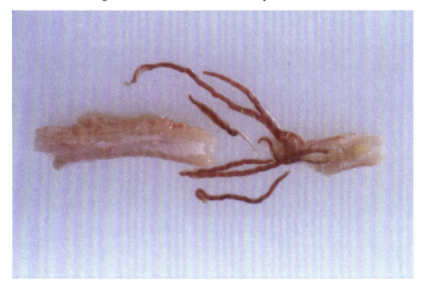

Syngamus trachea worms from a trachea

Syngamus trachea is a red worm with male and female forms. The female (around 2cm in length) is much larger than the male (0.5 cm), which is permanently attached to the female in copulation, forming a characteristic 'Y' shape. The eggs are carried up the trachea by the action of the excess mucous produced in response to the presence of the adults, and is then swallowed. The egg then passes in the faeces.

The next host can be infected by either ingesting the egg containing the larvae, ingesting the hatched larvae or by eating a transport host such as an earthworm, slug, snail or insect containing the hatched larvae. The ingested larvae penetrate the intestines of the bird and pass via the blood circulation to the lungs. There the larvae moults twice within approximately five days and moves up the bronchi to the trachea. The adult worms possess a large but shallow mouth with teeth at the base with which they attach themselves to the mucosa of the trachea. The eggs can survive for nearly a year in soil, and the hatched larvae can survive in an infective state within a transport host for several years.

The affects of this parasite are the physical blockage of the trachea, and pneumonia set up by the presence and migration of the larvae through the lung tissue.

ASCARIDS

Ascarids are helminth parasites of domestic and wild birds. Three species are discussed here, ***Ascaridia galli*** (poultry), ***A.dissimilis*** (turkeys) and ***A.columbae*** (pigeons.). These are white intestinal roundworms with male and female forms that are not considered to be highly pathogenic to birds. The females can attain a length of up to 12 cm.

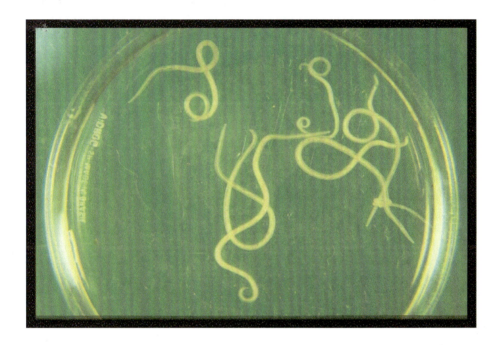

Ascaridia galli

The oval eggs are passed in the faeces, becoming infective after approximately three weeks. When ingested the larvae are released from the eggs and enter the intestinal mucosa where they can cause enteritis. In heavy infections this enteritis can become haemorrhagic.

In normal infections the presence of the adult worms can be undetected, in severe infections the combination of numbers and the large size of the worms can lead to intestinal blockage and mortality. Ascarid infection can also lower the host immunity to other infections such as Infectious Bronchitis

The severity of infection is proportional to the number of eggs ingested; the adult worms mate and produce eggs that become infective only after being voided from the host.

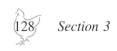

CAPILLARIA

Capillaria spp, also known as thread or hairworms are roundworms 1-5cm in length, which affect the crop and intestines of poultry. Three are considered important, as their pathogenic affects on the host when present in large numbers are far more serious than the larger Ascarid worms. These worms have male and female forms, the males being smaller in length than the females, the latter of which produce characteristic 'barrel' shaped eggs.

The worms bury their heads into the mucosa of their predilection sites, in heavy infestations this can lead to a diphtheric inflammation which, if severe can result in the membrane sloughing off. The presence of these worms can cause emaciation, reduced growth rate and lowered egg production, studies have shown that these effects can occur even in light infections of fewer than 100 worms.

There are three main species of Capillaria affecting birds:

Capillaria contorta.
Capillaria caudinflata.
Capillaria obsingata.

C.contorta and *C.caudinflata* require an intermediate host (earthworms), the ingestion of these vectors completing their lifecycle, and are therefore controllable in modern indoor rearing systems. *C.obsingata* has a direct lifecycle and can occur indoors in deep litter houses.

Capillaria contorta also known as *Capillaria annulatus* affects the oesophagus and crop of chickens, turkeys, ducks and wild birds. *Capillaria obsingata* also known as *(Baruscapillaria obsignata)* and *Capillaria caudinflata* affect the small intestine of chickens and turkeys with *C.caudinflata* also affecting the small intestine of pigeons.

The lesions produced by *Capillaria spp* are not characteristic, diagnosis tends to be made by microscopic examination of mucosal scrapings, however splitting the intestine, crop or oesophagus and placing it in a glass jar of water allows for rapid diagnosis when the worms stand out like the fringe of a rug when the jar is held up to the light.

Affected parts should be rejected as unfit for human consumption, if the carcase shows signs of systemic disturbance such as emaciation, the entire carcase and offal should be rejected due to the effects of extensive parasitism.

ECTOPARASITES

Ectoparasites, or parasites which live on the host's body, for the purposes of poultry meat inspection consists of two classes, insects, including flies, lice and fleas, and arachnids such as mites and ticks.

The main affect of the presence of ectoparasites on the host is one of irritation due to their presence; however, anaemia due to blood/fluid loss as well as drop in egg production can also be caused by these parasites. As with all parasitic infections, either internal or external, the opportunity for secondary bacterial infection is always a possibility. Most mites and lice are passed on by direct contact, although some such as fleas and the red mite are environmental parasites, which live in an area, and parasitize birds placed within that area. The role of wild birds, especially pigeons, in the transmission of Ectoparasites of poultry should not be underestimated, especially with the re-emerging popularity of free-range and organic rearing methods

INSECTS

Insects have three pairs of legs, with distinct head, thorax and abdomen and a pair of antennae.

Fleas

Echidnophaga gallinacea. (**The burrowing flea.**) produces nodules on the skin of poultry, commonly the wattles and comb, where the fertilised female burrows into the skin and lays eggs. When hatched, the larvae leave the nodules and drop to the ground. The larvae moult twice before forming a cocoon from which the adult emerges. The adult fleas are permanent inhabitants of the bird.

Ceratophyllus gallinae. (**Poultry Flea**), is a common flea infesting birds, and the commonest affecting poultry, and can cause severe anaemia, irritation and death. This flea can spend the majority of its lifecycle off the host, only needing to feed as an adult every 6 months as a minimum.

Lice

Menacanthus stramineus. (**Body Lice**). The body louse is a pale yellow-brown biting louse, up to 3mm in length and is possibly the most pathogenic of the 40 plus species of lice that can affect birds. The lifespan is approximately 1 month during which the female produces 200-300 eggs glued to the feathers (nits.) The eggs hatch to expose nymphs, a miniature version of the adult, which moult three times within 2-3 weeks to produce an adult. The adults are able to bite and chew, which enables them to eat feathers and down as well as skin scales. *M. stramineus* is found mostly in the areas of the anus, the thighs and the breast. The presence of this louse causes severe irritation and dermatitis, and can lead to anaemia through the feeding habit of puncturing feathers to feed on blood, as well as eating growing feather sheaths. Birds can cause damage to themselves by feather picking and scratching.

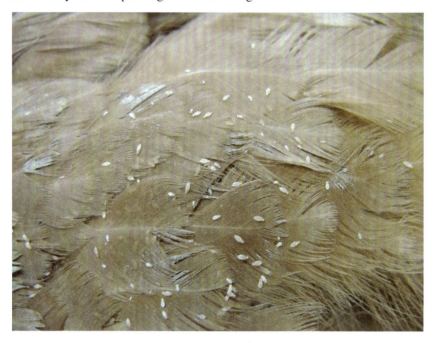

Menacanthus stramineus – unfed lice leaving a dead bird

Arachnids

Arachnid adults have four pairs of legs, there are no antennae, and the body is divided into a head/thorax and abdomen

Mites

Cnemidocoptes mutans. (Scaly leg mite) and *C.gallinae* (**depluming itch mite),** are the only burrowing mites of poultry, with a similar lifecycle to the *Sarcoptes spp* found in other mammals. The fertilised females feeding on the fluid from damaged sub dermal tissues as it forms tunnels in which it lays the eggs. The larvae produced burrow into the sub dermis and form pockets in which they moult to form into adults. The adults emerge through the skin and fertilise the females, repeating the lifecycle of around 20 days.

    C. mutans burrows into the skin beneath the scales on the legs, producing characteristic lesions of raised, ragged leg scales. *C.gallinae* burrows into feather shafts, prompting the host to pluck and remove the affected feathers to prevent the pain and irritation caused by the presence of the mite.

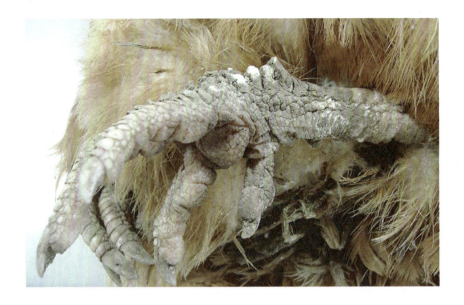

Scaley leg due to the action of *Cnemidocoptes mutans*

Dermanyssus gallinae (**the Red Mite**) is approximately 1.5mm in length and is a white to grey colour until full of blood. This mite only parasitises the host to feed nocturnally. The adults live and lay eggs in crevices in poultry houses, and both the nymphs and adults feed on blood, heavy infestations can cause severe anaemia, even death.

Laminosioptes cysticola. (**the Tissue mite**) forms nodules up to 2-3mm in diameter in muscles, internal viscera and the lungs. These nodules contain groups of mites, but due to their yellowish colouration and the usual calcification that occurs, these nodules can be confused with those of avian tuberculosis.

Ornithonyssus sylvarium. (**Northern Fowl Mite**), this species spends almost its entire life on the host; survival away from the host is limited to 10-20 days. The usual signs in the live bird are a blackened vent area due to large deposits of mite eggs.

NEOPLASIA

NEOPLASIA

INTRODUCTION

The term tumour literally applies to any abnormal swelling, but nowadays it tends to refer exclusively to neoplasms, which are abnormal new growth of tissue, in which cell multiplication is uncontrolled and progressive in addition to serving no purpose and growing faster than normal tissue. These neoplastic formations are classified as being either benign or malignant, the gross appearance of neoplasia is variable being dependant on their origin and type. Both malignant and benign tumours are served by increased blood vascularisation, any tumour requiring nutrients to continue growth. In the case of the rapidly growing malignant tumours the blood vessels tend to be thin, poorly formed and prone to rupture creating the appearance of haemorrhagic areas within the tumour.

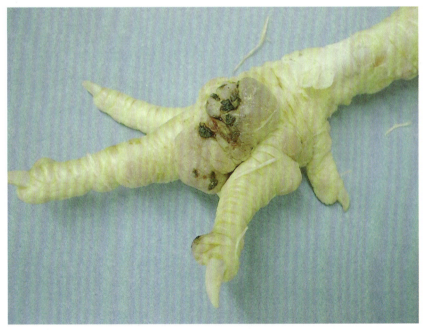

Tumour formation on the foot of a broiler

BENIGN TUMOURS

These grow slowly, pushing aside normal tissue without invading it. They are usually encapsulated and do not normally produce secondary tumours within the body. Although some benign tumours are caused by viruses, on the whole they do not appear to be infectious. The effect of their presence tends to be physical, blockage of systems in the body and pressure applied to organs being obvious examples.

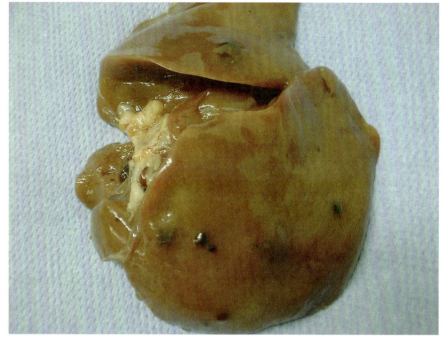

Hepatic haemangiomas – benign congenital of blood capillaries

Malignant tumours grow in an irregular shape and so quickly that the cell nutrition can become affected leading to cell death (necrosis) and ulceration. Malignant tumours invade surrounding tissue and can produce secondary tumours within the body through a process of metastasis (cells transported

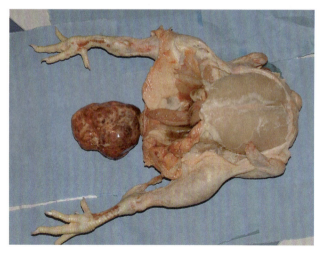

A malignant intestinal tumour

through the blood stream or lymphatic system), as well as through direct contact with other organs

Tumours in poultry are commonly malignant and caused by viral agents, differentiation between benign and malignant tumours is difficult to achieve in the abattoir.

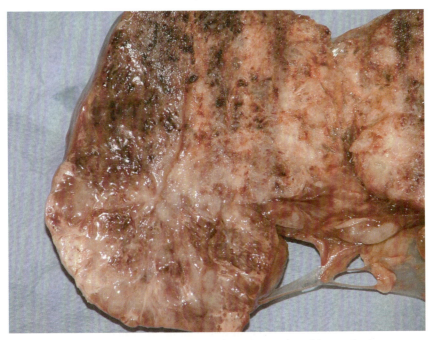

Incision into malignant tumour – variegated, necrotic and haemorrhagic

METASTASIS

This is the method of dissemination of malignant neoplasia throughout the body forming secondary tumours, the transfer of tumour cells tending to be either through direct contact between adjacent surfaces (contact spread) or via the blood or lymphatic circulation. Metastasis occurs as a product of the invasive abilities of malignant neoplasia, the detachment of tumour cells from the unencapsulated mass followed by infiltration of cells into surrounding tissue (contact), or erosion of the epithelial cells lining the blood and lymph vessels allowing ingress into the circulation. Studies have shown however that less than 1 in 10,000 neoplastic cells that enter these circulations will produce metastatic growth. As a general rule of thumb sarcomas are spread via the blood circulation and carcinomas via the lymphatics.

CHARACTERISTICS OF NEOPLASIA

Benign Tumours	Malignant Tumours
Grow slowly	Rapid growth
Usually encapsulated	Unencapsulated
Do not invade local tissue	Highly invasive
No metastatic spread	Metastatic spread
Cut surface bland and homogenous	Variegated, haemorrhage and necrosis

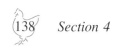

Infections that promote tumour formation in poultry include:

AVIAN LEUKOSIS

Synonyms	Big liver disease
Aetiology	RNA tumour **oncornovirus**. Three forms: Erythroid leukosis, Myeloid leukosis and Lymphoid leukosis.
Pathogenesis	Horizontal transmission by direct contact between chickens where the virus is present in saliva and faeces can occur but is rare due to short survival span of the virus in the environment. More often spread due to vertical transmission from the egg. Tumours initially develop in the Bursa, these can regress due to the action of the immune system as occurs in horizontally spread infection, or can metastasise to other organs, especially in the vertically transmitted form, where antibodies are not produced against the virus as those birds that are egg-infected become virally tolerant to this virus.
Gross lesions	**Erythroid** – Cherry red liver and spleen. Viraemia produces variable anaemia due to number of immature red blood cells in blood. **Myeloid** – Extra vascular neoplasms, the liver and spleen take on a 'Moroccan leather' appearance. Discreet nodular tumours with a chalky/cheesy consistency form. These have a predilection for the inner surfaces of the flat bones such as the internal surfaces of the ribs, pelvis and sternum. **Lymphoid** – Gross enlargement of the liver, tumours in spleen, gonads, kidney and in the intrafollicular areas of the bursa.
Judgement	Carcase and offal are unfit for human consumption.
Other information.	**Avian leukosis forms B-cell neoplasia. Generally in birds 16 weeks+.**

LYMPHOPROLIFERATIVE DISEASE OF TURKEYS

Synonyms	LPD
Aetiology	**Retrovirus**
Pathogenesis	Most common in turkeys between 10-18 weeks of age. Spread by direct contact between infected/non-infected birds.
Clinical signs	Dullness, lameness, partial paralysis is nerve involvement.
Gross lesions	Severe splenomegaly. If the liver is affected, it can become enlarged and contain pinpoint white lymphoid tumours. Microscopic infection of peripheral nerves more common than macroscopic enlargement.
Judgement	Carcase and offal unfit for human consumption.

MAREK'S DISEASE

Synonyms	Fowl paralysis, Floppy Broiler Syndrome, Range Paralysis, Polyneuritis, Neurolymphomatosis gallinarum.
Aetiology	Cell associated DNA virus of the **Herpes virus** group, with a predilection for peripheral nerves.
Pathogenesis	Mostly airborne transmission, virus replicates in feather follicle epithelial cells to form the enveloped fully infective particle and is therefore present in dander, dust and litter. In litter the virus can remain active for over a year. There are three stages in MD infection, Productive/Restrictive infection that results in B-cell death due to antigen infection, Latent Infection in T-cells (carrier state), and T-cell multiplication to form lymphoid neoplasia. Four forms of Marek's disease. Nervous, Visceral, Skin and Ocular. All may be present at the same time.
Clinical signs	**Occular form**- known as 'pearl eye, leads to partial or complete blindness as lymphocytic infiltrations produce an irregular pupil shape and irresponsiveness to light and greying of the iris. **Neural form**-classical Marek's affects peripheral nerves producing spastic paralysis of the wings and legs if the brachial and sciatic nerves are affected. A characteristic sign is birds unable to stand, lying with one leg extended forward, the other back. Other signs are dependant on the nerve groups inflamed; cervical nerves produce torticollis, intestinal nerves produce weight loss and diarrhoea, and affection of the vagus and intercostals nerves can lead to respiratory paralysis and death.
Gross lesions	**Nervous form** – Enlargement of peripheral nerves (2-3X) that lose their normal striations and white colouration. **Visceral form** – Diffuse, soft grey lymphomas and enlargement of organs such as the liver, gonads, spleen, lungs, proventriculus and heart. **Skin form** – Lymphomas of the skin and feather follicles.
Judgement	Carcase and offal unfit for human consumption.
Other information	T-cell neoplasia. Generally occurs around 6 weeks of age.

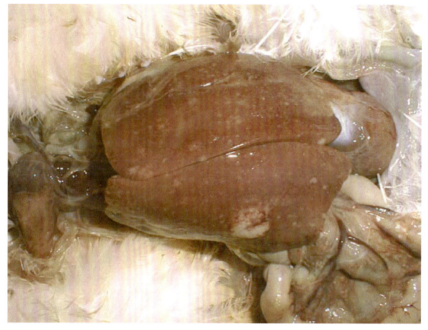

Mareks disease – liver from commercial broiler

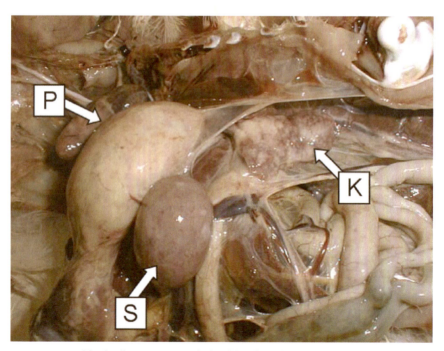

Mareks disease – proventriculus (P), spleen (S) and kidney (K)

Squaemous cell carcinoma – also known as Avian Keratoacanthoma, this is a malignant tumour of the epidermis, of uncertain aetiology, producing crater-like ulcers on the skin that can coalesce to form large lesions. Carcase and offal are unfit for human consumption.

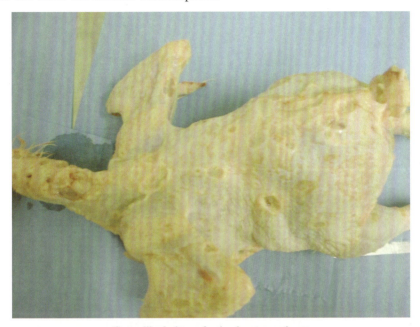

Crater-like lesions of avian keratoacanthoma

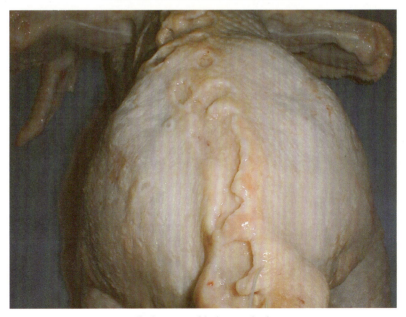

Coalescence of lesions on back

5

AFFECTIONS OF SPECIFIC PARTS

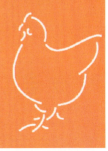

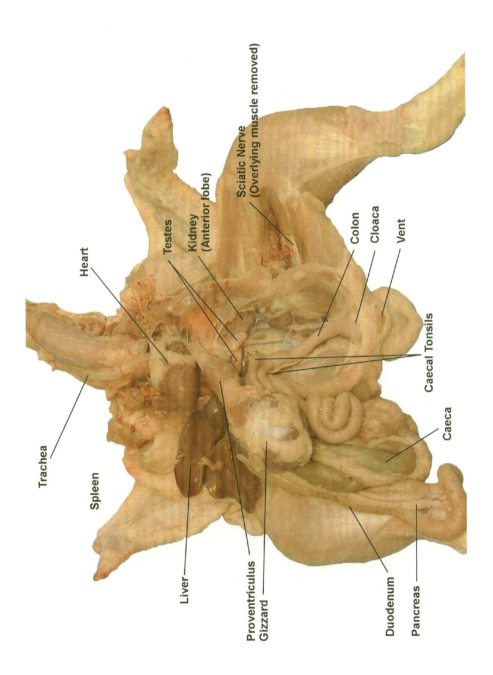

Heart

Testes

Kidney
(Anterior lobe)

Sciatic Nerve
(Overlying muscle removed)

Colon

Cloaca

Vent

Caecal Tonsils

Caeca

Trachea

Spleen

Liver

Proventriculus
Gizzard

Duodenum

Pancreas

Broiler – Internal Organ Map

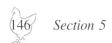

AFFECTIONS OF SPECIFIC PARTS

AIRSACS

LESIONS	POSSIBLE DIAGNOSIS
Inflammation of	Airsacculitis
Cloudy	Airsacculitis, infectious coryza, laryngotracheitis, influenza, Newcastle disease.
Foam, frothy	Infectious bronchitis
Mouldy, nodules	Aspergillosis
Foam, pus, thickened	Airsacculitis, colibacillosis, fowl cholera, Newcastle disease, chronic respiratory disease (CRD)

BODY CAVITY

LESIONS	POSSIBLE DIAGNOSIS
Straw coloured fluid	Ascites
Milky fluid	Peritonitis
Blood clot	Aortic rupture, Hepatic rupture
Petechial haemorrhages in abdominal fat	Avian influenza, toxaemia
Chalky deposits on serosal surfaces	Visceral gout
'Cooked' egg yolk	Egg peritonitis
Black, foul smelling pus	Traumatic peritonitis

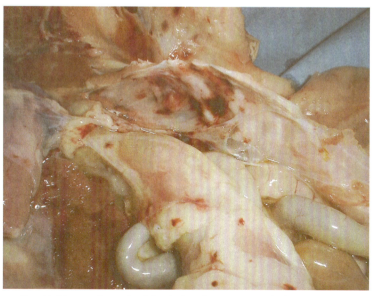

Petechial haemorrhages in abdominal cavity, on proventriculus and gizzard

CAECA

LESIONS	POSSIBLE DIAGNOSIS
Inflammation of	Typhlitis
Cores bloody or hard	Caecal coccidiosis
Small threadlike pieces	Caecal worms
Cores white	Coccidiosis, blackhead
Ulcers	Ulcerative enteritis

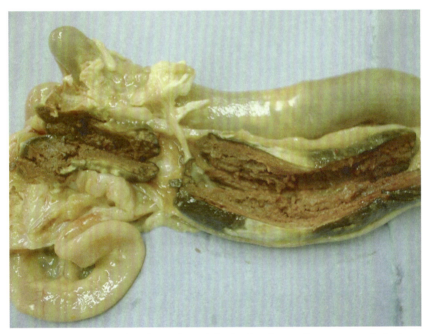

Caecal impaction – distension and containing hardened cores. Lower caecum incised

CLOACAL BURSA

LESIONS	POSSIBLE DIAGNOSIS
Inflammation of	Bursitis
Notably enlarged Atrophy	Infectious bursal disease (Gumboro) Non-specific infection Infectious bursal disease, Chicken anaemia virus

CROP

LESIONS	POSSIBLE DIAGNOSIS
Sour contents	Bluecomb disease
Towelling effect	Candidiasis
Distended, full of rancid material	Crop impaction, pendulous crop
White cheesy growth	Moniliasis

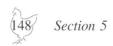

DROPPINGS

LESIONS	POSSIBLE DIAGNOSIS
Brown, foamy, intermittent	Caecal droppings
Diarrhoea	Enteritis
Haemorrhagic	Coccidiosis, Newcastle Disease
Bright yellow	Blackhead
Light yellow/yellow-green	Typhoid, Fowl cholera
Constantly foamy	Protozoal parasitism
Poorly digested feed	Infectious stunting syndrome

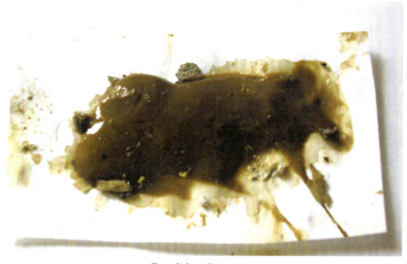

Caecal droppings

FEET

LESIONS	POSSIBLE DIAGNOSIS
Immobile joints	Tenosynovitis
Swollen foot pad	Infectious Synovitis, articular gout, tenosynovitis, bumblefoot
Blackened, crusty foot pad	Pododermatitis,
Deep ulceration	Plantar necrosis

GIZZARD

LESIONS	POSSIBLE DIAGNOSIS
Erosion of cutica gastrica	Necrotic enteritis, enteritis, haemorrhagic anaemia
Cutica gastrica will not peel	Necrotic enteritis
Excess fibre, grit etc	Impaction

HEAD

LESIONS	POSSIBLE DIAGNOSIS
Swollen, puffy	Infectious coryza, Newcastle disease, Injury. Swollen head syndrome, cellulitis
Nodules on comb	Fowl pox
White, scaly, powdery comb	Favus
Watery eyes	Infectious coryza, trauma
Blindness	Fowl pox, Aspergillosis, Paracolon, paratyphoid, ammonia blindness.
Watery, red, inflamed	Newcastle disease, laryngotracheitis, ammonia burn
Irregular pupil, pearl eye	Marek's disease
Eye enlarged, swollen	Mycoplasma infection
Face swollen	Infectious coryza, Newcastle disease, *E.coli,* swollen head syndrome
Darkened, purplish	Erysipelas, septicaemia, fowl cholera, injury
Nasal discharge	Infectious coryza, CRD, Infectious bronchitis, Influenza
Wattles swollen, bulbous	Infectious coryza, fowl cholera

HEART

LESIONS	POSSIBLE DIAGNOSIS
Inflammation of surrounding sac	Pericarditis
Inflammation of surface	Epicarditis
Inflammation of cardiac muscle	Myocarditis
Inflammation of internal surface	Endocarditis
Pericardium thickened, fibrinous, yellowing	Colibacillosis, chronic respiratory disease, fowl cholera, avian chlamydiosis
Hydropericardium	Ascites, Aflatoxin, poisoning,
Haemorrhages	Fowl cholera, typhoid, erysipelas, haemorrhagic anaemia
Necrotic foci	Pullorum
Heart enlarged	Ascites, Round Heart Disease
Vegetative endocarditis	Amyloidosis

INTESTINES

LESIONS	POSSIBLE DIAGNOSIS
Inflammation of	Enteritis
White roundworms	*Ascaridia galli*
Pin point haemorrhages	Coccidiosis
Red and white dots	Coccidiosis (*E. necatrix*)

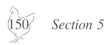

Granulomas	Colibacillosis (Hjärre's disease), tumours.
Reddening	Non-specific enteritis
Bloody	Coccidiosis (*E. necatrix*), Newcastle disease
Small white strips	Coccidiosis
Thickened, swollen, haemorrhagic	Enteritis, coccidiosis
Annular bands	Duck virus enteritis
Red circular patches	Haemopoetic foci

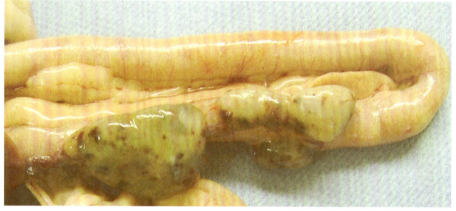

Neoplasia on the duodenum

KIDNEYS

LESIONS	POSSIBLE DIAGNOSIS
Inflammation of	Nephritis
Swollen, urate deposit	Gout, Nephrosis, Gumboro, Infectious bronchitis
Mottled	Nephrosis, infectious bronchitis, inclusion body hepatitis

LEGS

LESIONS	POSSIBLE DIAGNOSIS
Inflammation of joints	Arthritis
Inflammation of tendons	Tendonitis
Inflammation of tendon and sheath	Tenosynovitis
Bones thickened, enlarged	Lymphoid leukosis, tenosynovitis, osteopetrosis
Joint swelling	Synovitis, paratyphoid, pullorum, arthritis, tenosynovitis.
Cap separated from head of femur	Femoral epiphysiolysis, Femoral head necrosis
White, pasty material in joints	Articular gout
Green discolouration of thigh tissue	Ruptured gastrocnemius tendon
Paralysis	Marek's disease, Botulism, Spondylolisthesis, heat stroke, Cage Layer Fatigue, Acute dehydration, Nutritional deficiency
Exterior rough and scaly	Scaly Leg mite, Fowl pox

Displacement of gastrocnemius tendon	Perosis
Persistant plug of cartilage beneath growth plate	Tibial dyschondroplasia
Haemorrhages	Avian influenza (HP)

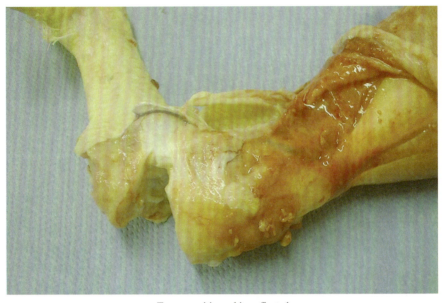

Tenosynovitis – skin reflected

LIVER

LESIONS	POSSIBLE DIAGNOSIS
Inflammation of	Hepatitis
Inflammation of capsule	Perihepatitis
Perihepatitis	Chronic respiratory disease, colibacillosis, fowl cholera
Mottling and necrosis	Vibronic hepatitis, inclusion body hepatitis, chicken anaemia virus
White or yellow foci	Fowl cholera, hepatitis, pullorum, ulcerative enteritis, adenovirus infection, pasteurellosis, ulcerative enteritis
Swollen, darkened	Fowl cholera, typhoid, erysipelas, septicaemia, toxaemia, inclusion body hepatitis.
Creamy sandy foci	Avian tuberculosis, pseudotuberculosis
Enlarged, firm and pale	Lymphoid leukosis, Marek's disease
Large creamy nodules	Lymphoid leukosis
Green discolouration,	Hepatitis, staphylococcal infection, blockage of bile ducts, infectious synovitis
Bronze colour and enlarged	Fowl typhoid
Yellowish discolouration	Fatty liver syndrome, aflatoxicosis, septicaemia

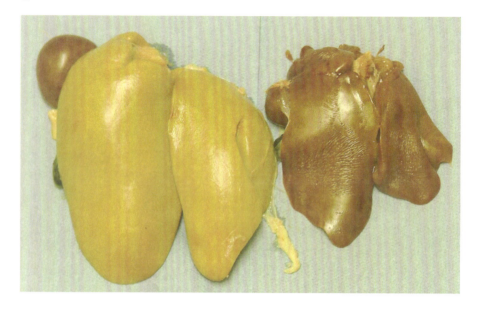

A 'fatty liver' from a septicaemic carcase on left compared with average sample from same flock. (Note the enlargement of the spleen)

LUNGS

LESIONS	POSSIBLE DIAGNOSIS
Inflammation of	Pneumonia
Consolidated	Pneumonia
Congestion	Aspiration contamination, anatipestifer, badly bled,
Yellow/cream nodules	Aspergillosis, pasteurellosis, pullorum

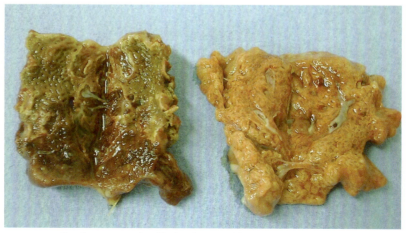

Purulent pneumonia affecting lung on left. Both samples incised

OVARIES AND OVIDUCT

LESIONS	POSSIBLE DIAGNOSIS
Inflammation of oviduct	Salpingitis
Vegetative growth	Marek's disease
Broken egg yolks	Fowl cholera, infectious bronchitis
Distension and containing partly formed eggs	Impaction of the oviduct
Follicles hard and shrunken	Pullorum, typhoid
Caseous exudate in oviduct	Impaction, salpingitis

PROVENTRICULUS

LESIONS	POSSIBLE DIAGNOSIS
Inflammation of	Proventriculitis, Gastritis
Swollen, enlarged	Necrotic enteritis, Infectious Stunting Syndrome
Haemorrhagic	Newcastle disease, Chicken anaemia virus

SKIN

LESIONS	POSSIBLE DIAGNOSIS
Inflammation of	Dermatitis
Nodules, mainly legs	Marek's disease
Moist, necrotic patches	Exudative diathesis, Gangrenous / Necrotic dermatitis
Crusted areas	Erysipelas, scab, Gangrenous dermatitis.
Green discolouration	Bruising, Gangrenous dermatitis.
Vent irritation	Northern fowl mite, Vent gleet, vices.
Darkened, purplish	Erysipelas, Fowl cholera
Crater like lesions	Squaemous cell carcinoma
Congestion and petechial haemorrhages	Avian influenza, toxaemia, uncut

SPLEEN

INFLAMMATION OF	SPLENITIS
Enlargement	Splenomegaly
Granulomatous lesions	Avian tuberculosis
Splenomegaly	Fowl typhoid, infectious synovitis
Splenomegaly and mottling	Inclusion body hepatitis, marble spleen disease (pheasants), pasteurellosis, pullorum
Atrophy	Chicken anaemia virus,
Splenomegaly and rupture	Amyloidosis, trauma, toxaemia

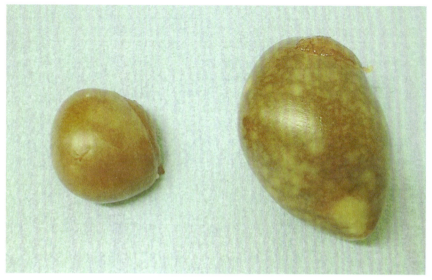

Splenomegaly and mottling of spleen on right compared to normal

TRACHEA

LESIONS	POSSIBLE DIAGNOSIS
Inflammation of	Tracheitis
Red Y-shaped threads	*Syngamus trachea*
Haemorrhagic mucous	Chronic respiratory disease
Nodules	Fowl pox
Diphtheric membrane	Fowl pox
Free blood or pus-like lining	Newcastle disease, laryngotracheitis
Cheese-like plug	Infectious laryngotracheitis

DISEASE AND CAUSE

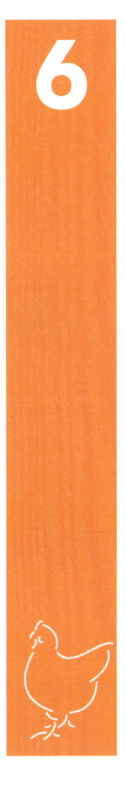

6

DISEASE	CAUSE	TYPE
Anatipestifer (New Duck Disease, Infectious serositis)	*Pasteurella anatipestifer*	Bacterial
Ascaridiasis	*Ascaridia galli* (poultry) *A.dissimilis* (turkeys) *A.columbae* (pigeons)	Parasitic
Aspergillosis (Brooder Pneumonia, Mycotic pneumonia, Pneumomycosis)	*Aspergillus flavus* *Aspergillus fumigatus*	Fungal
Avian Chlamydiosis (Ornithosis, Psitticosis)	*Chlamydia psittaci*	Rickettsiae
Avian Influenza (Fowl Plague)	Orthomyxovirus	Viral
Avian Leukosis (Big Liver Disease)	Oncornovirus	Viral
Avian Mycoplasmosis (Chronic Respiratory Disease) (Infectious Synovitis)	*Mycoplasma gallisepticum* *Mycoplasma meleagridis* *Mycoplasma synoviae*	Bacterial
Avian Salmonellosis (Paratyphoid)	*Salmonella spp* especially *Salmonella typhimurium*	Bacterial
Avian Tuberculosis	*Mycobacterium avium*	Bacterial
Blackhead	*Histomonas meleagridis*	Protozoal
Botulism (Limberneck, Western Duck Sickness)	*Clostridium botulinum*	Bacterial toxins
Caecal worm	*Heterakis gallinarum*	Parasitic
Candidiasis (Thrush, Moniliasis, Sour crop, Crop mycosis)	*Candida albicans*	Fungal
Capillaria	*Capillaria contorta* *Capillaria caudinflata* *Capillaria obsingata*	Parasitic
Chicken Anaemia Virus (Infectious Anaemia)	Circovirus	Viral
Coccidiosis	*Eimeria species*	Protozoal parasite

DISEASE	CAUSE	TYPE
Curled toe paralysis	Riboflavin deficiency	Nutritional
Duck Virus Enteritis (Duck Plague)	Herpesvirus	Viral
Duck Virus Hepatitis	Picornavirus	Viral
Erysipelas (Leatherhead)	*Erysipelothrix rhusiopathiae*	Bacterial
Exudative diathesis	Vitamin E deficiency	Nutritional
Favus (White Comb)	*Trichophyton meganinii*	Fungal
Fleas	*Echidnophaga gallinacea* (The burrowing flea) *Ceratophyllus gallinae* (Poultry Flea)	Parasitic
Fowl Pox (Avian Diphtheria, Contagious epithelioma)	Pox Virus	Viral
Fowl Typhoid	*Salmonella gallinarum*	Bacterial
Gangrenous Dermatitis (Avian Malignant Oedema)	*Clostridium septicum*	Bacterial
Gapes	*Syngamus trachea*	Parasitic
Goose Viral Hepatitis (Derszy's Disease)	Parvovirus	Viral
Haemorrhagic Enteritis of Turkeys	Adenovirus	Viral
Hexamitiasis	*Hexamita meleagridis*	Parasitic
Inclusion Body Hepatitis (Haemorrhagic anaemia syndrome)	Adenovirus	Viral
Infectious Bronchitis	Coronavirus	Viral
Infectious Bursal Disease (Gumboro, Infectious bursitis)	Birnavirus	Viral
Infectious Coryza	*Haemophilus gallinarum*	Bacterial
Infectious Laryngotracheitis	Herpes Virus	Viral
Infectious Stunting (Malabsorption Syndrome, infectious proventriculitis)	Reovirus	Viral

DISEASE	CAUSE	TYPE
Lice	*Menacanthus stramineus* (Body Lice)	Parasitic
Marble Spleen Disease (Lung Oedema)	Avian adenovirus	Viral
Marek's Disease (Fowl Paralysis)	Herpesvirus	Viral
Mycotoxicosis (Aflatoxicosis, Turkey X disease)	Fungal toxin	Fungal
Mites	*Cnemidocoptes mutans* (Scaly leg mite) *Cnemidocopte .gallinae* (deplumming itch mite) *Dermanyssus gallinae* (the Red Mite) *Laminosioptes cysticola* (the Tissue mite) *Ornithonyssus sylvarium* (Northern Fowl Mite)	Parasitic
Necrotic Enteritis (Cauliflower Gut, Rot gut)	*Clostridium perfringens*	Bacterial
Newcastle Disease (Fowl Pest)	Paramyxovirus	Viral
Paracolon Infection (Arizonosis)	*Arizona hinshawi*	Bacterial
Pasteurellosis (Fowl Cholera)	*Pasteurella multocida*	Bacterial
Perosis	Manganese deficiency	Nutritional
Pseudotuberculosis	*Yersinia pseudotuberculosis*	Bacterial
Pullorum Disease	*Salmonella pullorum*	Bacterial
Rickets	Vitamin D deficiency	Nutritional
Swollen head syndrome (Avian rhinotracheitis, 'Swellhead')	Pneumovirus	Viral
Trichomoniasis (Canker, Frounce)	*Trichomonas gallinarum* *Trichomonas columbae*	Parasitic
Transmissible Enteritis of Turkeys (Bluecomb)	Coronavirus	Viral

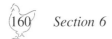

DISEASE	CAUSE	TYPE
Ulcerative Enteritis (Quail Disease)	*Clostridium colinum*	Bacterial
Viral Arthritis	Reovirus	Viral

7

CONDITIONS FOUND AT POST MORTEM INSPECTION IN ABATTOIRS

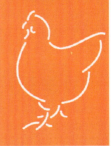

AIRSACCULITIS

The respiratory system is one of the five routes of infection into the body. The act of inspiration draws in pathogens that can then produce disease once the defences of the immune system of the body are overcome.

Most respiratory infections eventually produce lesions in the airsacs, these lesions tends to spread due to the lower vascularisation of these membranous sacs and therefore the reduced ability for the immune system to access the area.

Avian Mycoplasmosis tends to be the main cause of airsacculitis producing yellowish cloudiness of the airsacs that develops in time to thick pus. The respiratory system and especially the airsacs are also prone to secondary infection by pathogens such as *E.coli* once the immunity is lowered by the primary infection.

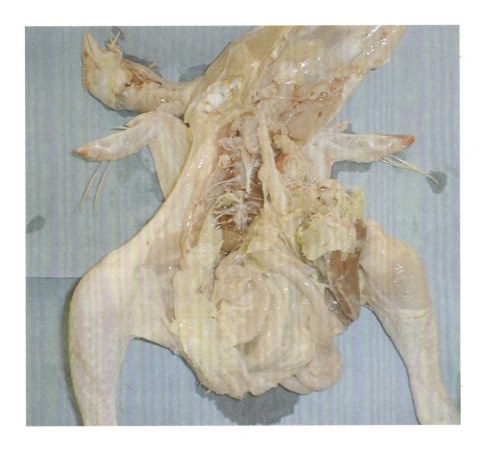

Chronic, purulent airsacculitis in a broiler

In cases of upper respiratory tract infections, the affected area should be rejected; if the carcase is emaciated or there are signs of systemic disturbance, the carcase and associated offal should be rejected as unfit for human consumption.

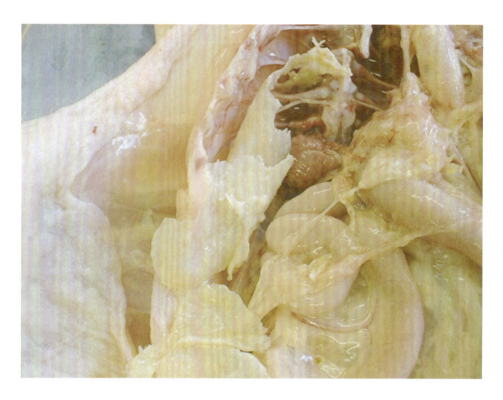

Detail of the lesions found in previous carcase

In the case of airsacculitis, judgement should be made according to the airsac affected and the form of exudate/inflammation present. In all cases where localised rejection is considered, the affected airsacs should be removed. If the clavicular airsac is affected, the humerus, deep pectoral muscle and neck should also be rejected.

If there is evidence of pericarditis or perihepatitis the entire carcase and offal should be rejected as unfit for human consumption.

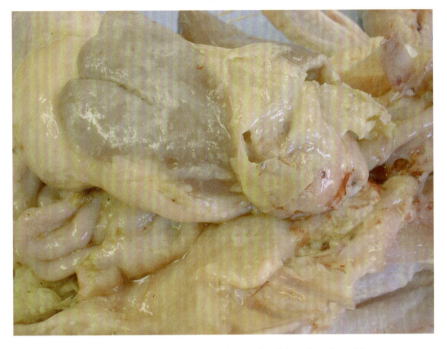

Airsacculitis associated with purulent pericarditis and perihepatitis.

ARTHRITIS/TENOSYNOVITIS

Inflammation of the joints, tendon sheaths and synovial membranes in poultry can be attributed to various factors such as reoviruses, *Mycoplasma synoviae*, bacterial infections and trauma. Most commonly affected are the tendons and sheaths associated with the hock joints, resulting in swelling, deformity and lameness. Incision of affected areas normally exposes inflamed, oedematous tendon sheaths with fibrinous deposits around the joint proper. In cases of *Mycoplasma synoviae* infection, the synovial fluid may contain exudates that become orangey-brown in the chronic infection.

Affected parts should be rejected, with the carcase examined to assess whether the infection is systemic or a rising infection from the feet. If the carcase is septicaemic or cachexic, the entire carcase and offal should be rejected as unfit for human consumption.

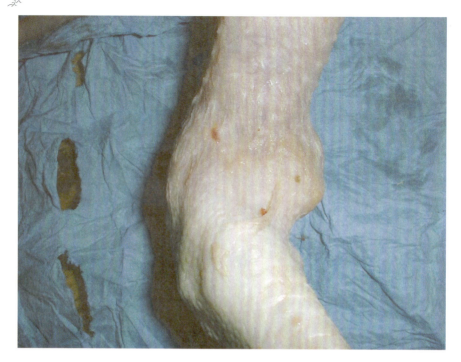

Typical post-mortem lesions, swelling of the hock joint with palpable exudates

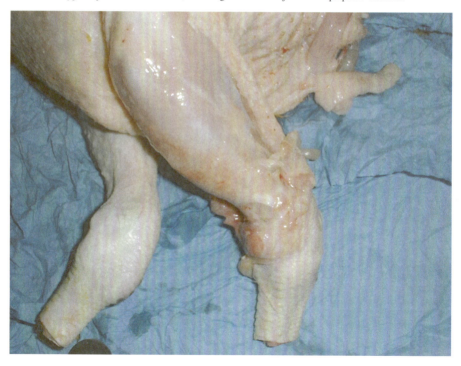

Bilateral tenosynovitis, skin reflected from one leg to expose fibrinous exudates and oedema of the surrounding tissue. Note petechial haemorrhaging above the lesion

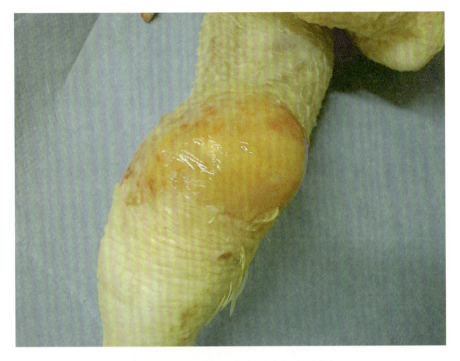

Mycoplasma synoviae infection of the hock joint

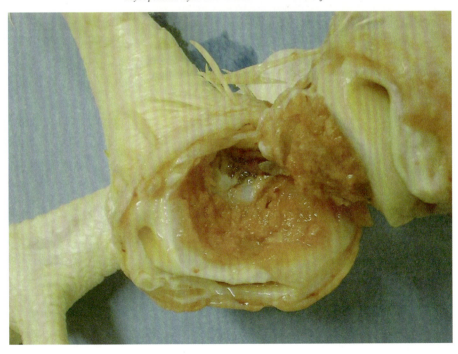

Incision into joint, revealing orangey-brown deposits indicative of chronic *Mycoplasma synoviae* infection

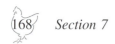
ASCITES / OEDEMA

Oedema is the abnormal accumulation of fluid within the body cavity and tissues. This fluid can collect in any part of the body, when present in a subcutaneous location it is known as anasarca; ascites when in the abdominal cavity (colloquially known as 'water-belly'); and hydropericardium when found in the pericardial sac.

HYDROPERICARDIUM / HAEMOPERICARDIUM

Dilation of the pericardium with clear or straw coloured fluid warrants rejection of the offal and judgement of the carcase on merits, and should not be confused with the fibrino-purulent lesions associated with *Salmonella enteriditis* infection.

Haemopericardium presents as a distended blood filled pericardial sac, usually due to rupture of one of the coronary arteries during the course of infection.

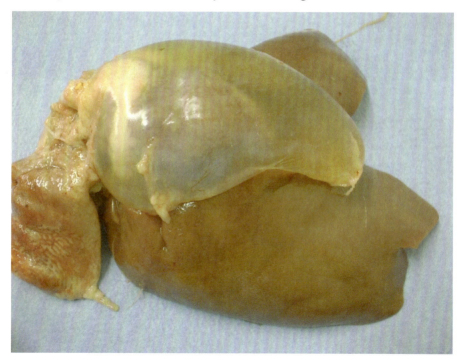

Hydropericardium

ANASARCA

The skin in poultry is loosely connected to the underlying tissues; therefore any condition affecting the subcutaneous area has the ability to spread.

Anasarca describes the accumulation of fluid in this subcutaneous area. In most cases this fluid accumulation takes on a jelly-like consistency due to the presence of fibrin.

Anasarca can occur in conjunction with Ascites but is most commonly encountered as a primary lesion. It tends to occur as a result of vascular damage due to the presence of toxins or due to dietary insufficiency such as exudative diathesis which occurs in cases of vitamin E deficiency. Usually anasarca in broilers is confined to the area of the wings and back, with an obvious fluid filled swelling in that area. Removal of the skin reveals straw coloured fluid or jelly. It is important to differentiate this condition from the aspiration of scald tank water.

Carcases displaying lesions consistent with anasarca should be rejected as unfit for human consumption.

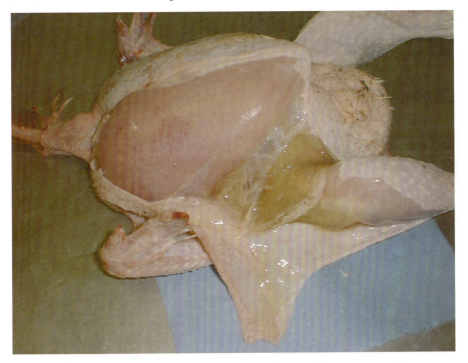

Anasarca – note gelatinous fluid and petechial haemorrhaging of the pectoral muscle

ASCITES

The term Ascites relates to an abnormal quantity of fluid in the abdominal spaces, this fluid most commonly collecting in the rear dorsal hepatic and intestinal spaces. In broilers the dorsal hepatic space is further divided by the post hepatic septum, and the quantity and condition of the fluid can vary on each side of this. The increase in fluid can be due to vascular damage, hepatic disruption (especially liver fibrosis), disturbance of the passage of lymph through the body as can occur in the presence of tumours; but is most commonly associated with a restriction of the blood flow through the lungs increasing the pressure of the pulmonary circulation (pulmonary hypertension) which in turn leads to dilation and failure of the right ventricle of the heart. This cardiac failure increases the blood pressure in both the liver and the blood circulation; causing the fluid component of the blood to leak out.

Ascites is more prevalent in poultry than in the red meat species mostly owing to the anatomy / physiology of the respiratory system. The lungs in broilers do not expand during respiration, the flow of air through them being dependant on the expansion of the airsacs. This lack of elasticity in the lung tissue leads to an inability on the part of the capillaries to expand to allow increased blood flow when a greater oxygen demand is placed on the system, this, in conjunction with the inflexibility of the nucleated red blood cells leads to pulmonary hypertension.

The high number of lesions encountered that suggest increased oxygen demand as a contributory factor, has led to the prevalence of ascites in a flock being considered an indicator of the environmental conditions during rearing on the farm, especially ventilation levels and carbon dioxide concentration.

At the wholebird inspection point the abdomen of the bird is distended with fluid, hence the colloquial term of 'water belly'.

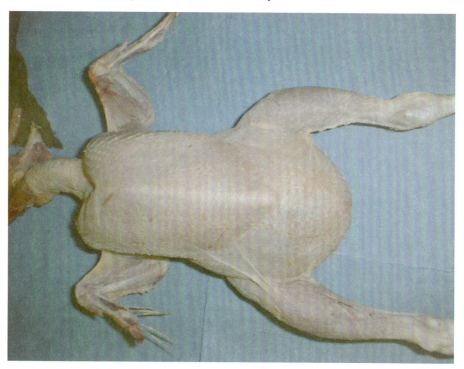

Distended fluid filled abdomen

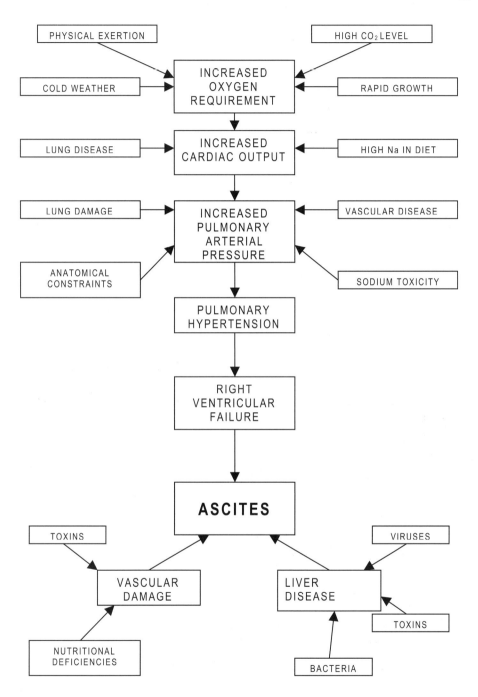

Summary of main causes of ascites

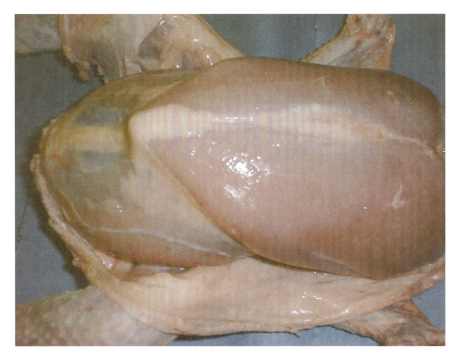

Ascitic carcase – skin reflected

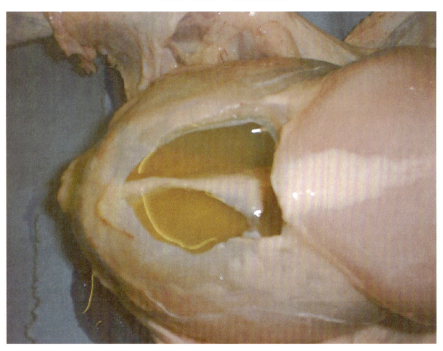

Incision through abdomen illustrating fluid collected and post-hepatic septum

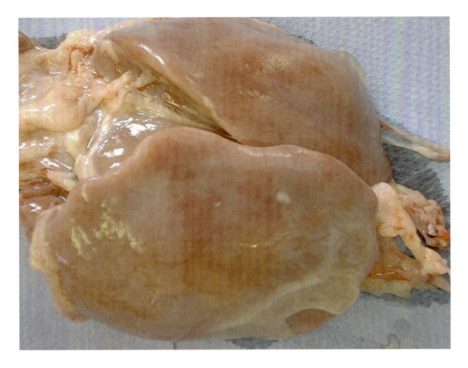

Liver lesions –described as pale, round edged and 'par boiled'

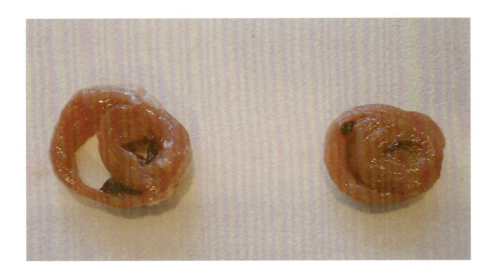

Right ventricular dilation of cross section of heart on left compared with normal on right

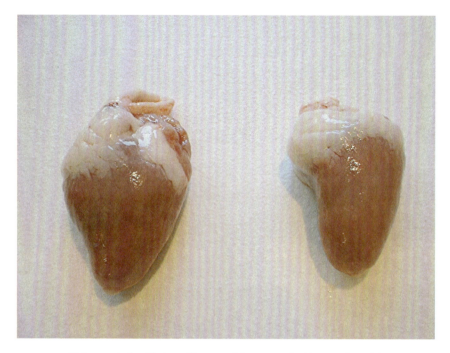

Right ventricular dilation of heart on left compared with normal on right

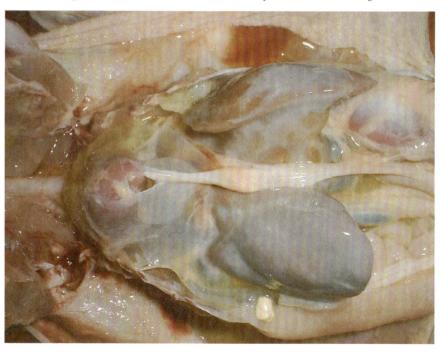

Ascites can also be associated with the formation of fibrin on surfaces, often with free floating clots accumulating within the ascitic fluid.

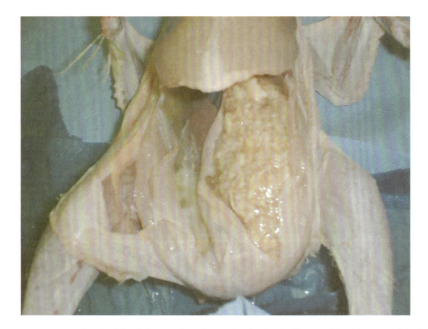

The separate nature of each side of the post-hepatic septum is clearly illustrated in this case, with clots of fibrin present on the left hand side cavity of the picture and purulent material in the right following secondary bacterial invasion.

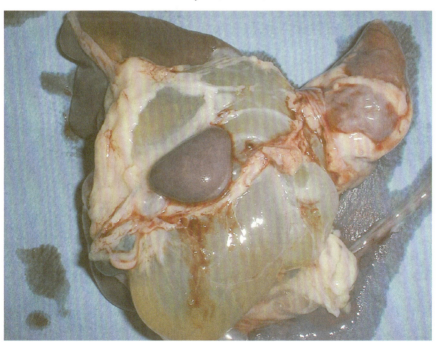

Sub-capsular hepatic oedema is a further common finding in cases of ascites when fluid accumulates under the visceral peritoneum of the liver

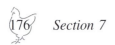

In cases of chronic ascites, the liver may appear cooked and have rounded edges; the straw-coloured ascitic fluid may contain flecks of blood and clots of fibrin; in addition there may be secondary bacterial infection with the formation of pus in the ascitic fluid.

Birds displaying lesions consistent with ascites/oedema should be rejected with their associated offal as unfit for human consumption. Although a background level of ascites is usually present in any flock, a higher percentage can be an indication of poor environmental conditions during the growing period.

BUMBLEFOOT

Bumblefoot is a bacterial infection of the plantar surface of the foot usually caused by *Staphylococcus aureus*, although other bacteria and factors such as fungi have been isolated from lesions. Unlike pododermatitis, which is almost a chemical burn causing necrosis of the dermis, bumblefoot is associated with a deeper infection producing calluses and hyperplastic tissue formation, culminating in the characteristic 'balling' of the foot.

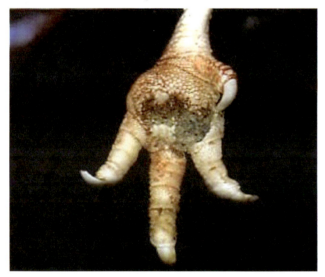

Bumblefoot of a turkey

This condition is more prevalent in heavier breeds such as turkeys, and in layers housed in percheries where damage to the footpad allows infection to develop. Chronic lesions can become ulcerated and extend into deeper tissues and joints, tenosynovitis of the tendons of the hock and feet being common in untreated cases.

Affected parts should be rejected. If there is evidence of systemic spread, such as septicaemia or emaciation, the entire carcase and offal should be rejected.

DEEP PECTORAL MYOPATHY
(Green Muscle Disease. Oregon Disease)

This is a non-infectious condition, whereby muscle degeneration and necrosis is caused by a combination of exertion and the physiology of the bird.

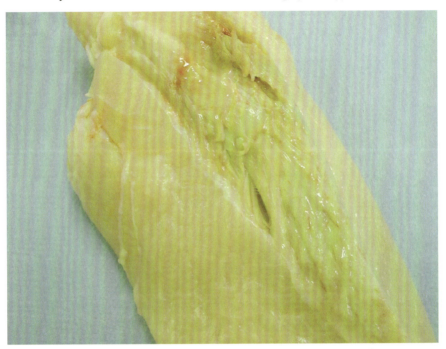

Oregon disease. Breast muscle removed from carcase to expose necrotic underlying fillet muscle.

The supracoracoideus muscle is enclosed in an inelastic membrane. During periods of intense muscular activity the muscles swell as the blood flow to them increases. The fascia constricts the enlargement of the supracoracoideus until the expanding muscle eventually constricts and then occludes its own blood supply. The swollen muscle is now unable to receive oxygen via the blood, nor release the trapped blood and the muscle cells die. This condition is known as an ischaemic myonecrosis, death of muscle cells due to deficiency of blood either through obstruction or functional constriction.

The supracoracoideus muscle initially becomes gelatinous and red resolving to a dry, greenish coloured mass. The lesion, as it is not due to pathological causes, is sterile, but does discolour to a brownish green on cooking and as such is not of the nature, substance or quality demanded by the consumer. This condition occurs more frequently in male turkeys where the lesions may be uni or bi-lateral. Dishing of the pectoral muscle over the lesion may be observed and in turkeys the insertion of a light source into the

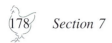

body cavity may reveal the lesion as a shadow due to the dense nature of the necrotic muscle.

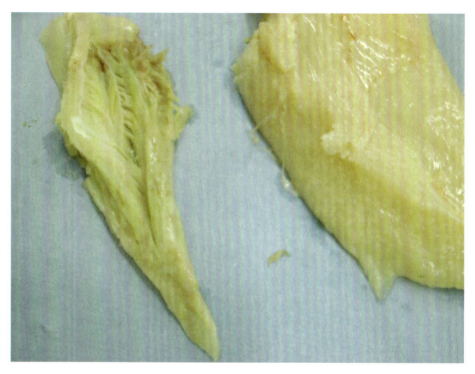

Deep pectoral myopathy. Supracoracoideus muscle removed and incised to show uniformity of colour, dry cooked appearance and unaffected pectoral muscle.

Affected muscle can be easily removed from the pectoral muscle, and should be rejected as unfit for human consumption.

EMACIATION / CACHEXIA

Cachexia and emaciation are conditions where body tissue regresses, particularly the breast muscles and body fat. **Cachexia** is defined as being wasting due to a pathological condition such as tuberculosis or avian chlamydiosis etc. **Emaciation** is defined as wasting due to malnutrition, true starvation, due to various reasons including the inability to reach food, as in cases of partial paralysis, for example spondylolisthesis. Both conditions are indistinguishable from each other at inspection. The sternum is very prominent due to wasting of the pectoral muscles. The fat deposits of the heart and abdomen are missing or are gelatinous. The breast muscles are dark, sticky and dehydrated. When pressed, the muscles do not spring back to their normal shape.

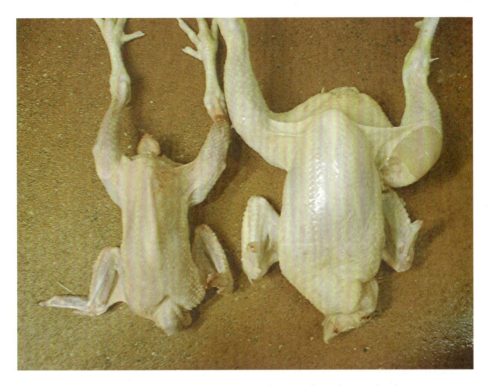

A cachexic bird compared with a normal carcase from the same batch.

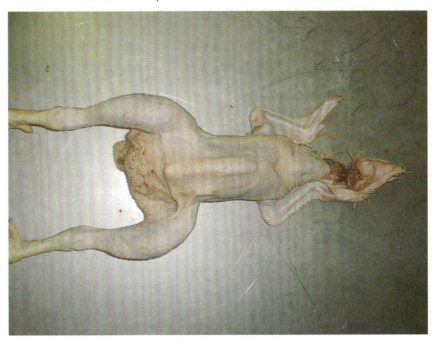

A bird rejected for emaciation / cachexia

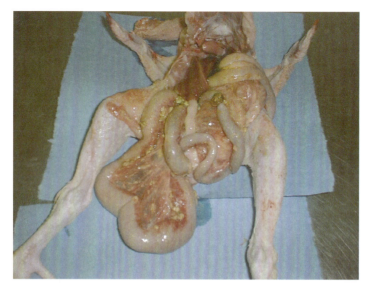

Incision into abdomen of previous carcase revealed purulent enteritis as the cause of the cachexia

Emaciated/cachexic carcases and associated offal are unfit for human consumption.

Biotin deficiency –a deficiency in available biotin can influence the percentage pododermatitis within a flock in addition to retardation of growth. Biologically available biotin is an essential nutrient for the maintenance of, amongst other things, epithelial tissue, particularly of the beak and the plantar surface of the foot, the latter of which is affected by deep fissures when a deficit of this nutrient occurs. The affect of the deficiency is also characterised by cachexia and lesions at the beak/skull junction leading to an increased number of 'parrot beaked' animals.

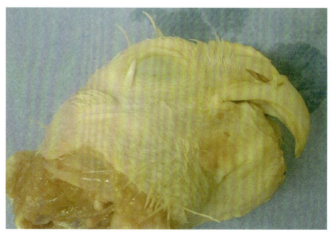

A typical 'parrot beaked' bird

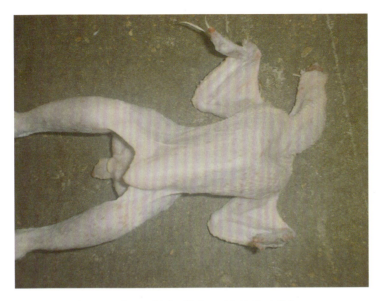

A carcase from a bird suffering with biotin deficiency

Runts, birds that are much smaller than the batch averages should be rejected at the point of hanging on. These birds should have been culled during the rearing period and not caught. The reasons for not hanging birds in this category is both the welfare risk to the animal in missing automated stunning equipment and cutters and due to the high contamination risk they pose in automated evisceration machinery.

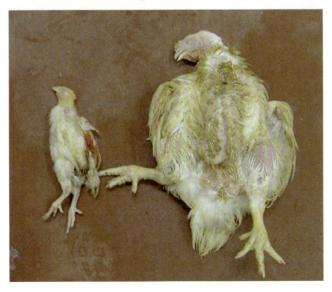

A runt compared with a normal bird from the same flock. Note the persistence of yellow down feathers on the head of the affected bird

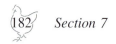

ENTERITIS

Enteritis is inflammation of the intestines. It can be either acute or chronic and occurs during the course of some diseases, or as a result of the action of parasites or toxic agents.

As ingestion is one of the five routes of infection into the body, inflammation of the digestive tract, especially the intestines is a common gross lesion of many conditions. The gross lesions encountered should be taken in context with other lesions in other organs of the body to reach a tentative basic diagnosis.

In making a decision, the health status of the other birds in the batch should be considered, for example, severe haemorrhage of the proventriculus and caecal tonsils within a batch can be indicative of viscerotropic velogenic Newcastle Disease and in ducks the presence of macroscopically visible annular bands of lymphoid tissue throughout the intestines is a characteristic lesion associated with Duck Virus Hepatitis.

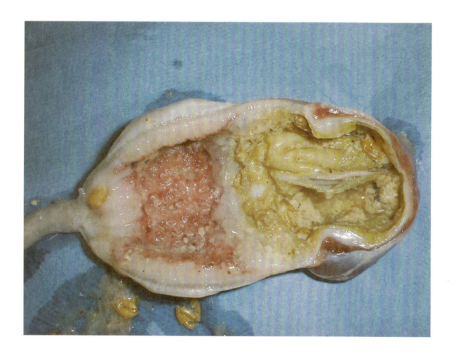

VVND – Haemorrhaging in the mucosa of the proventriculus

Enteritis can be non-specific, a reddening of the intestines with no obvious causal factor.

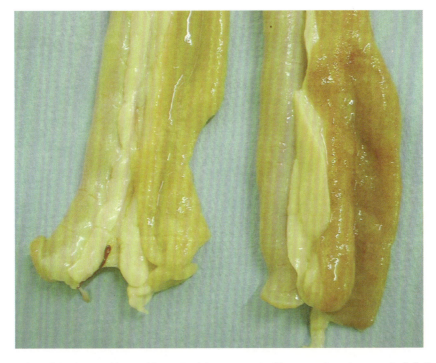

A section of duodenum with enteritis on the right, compared with a normal specimen on the left. Both samples have been partially incised to show lining. Note the hypertrophic pancreas of the affected sample.

Other characteristic forms of enteritis include:

Intestines distended, contents watery and foamy (gas) – acute bluecomb of turkeys.

Blood in intestines – haemorrhagic enteritis of turkeys, coccidiosis.

Button like ulcers -Quail's disease

Petechial haemorrhages-Fowl Cholera

Vegetative growths and foul smell associated with necrotic enteritis infections

Slimy enteritis due to Fowl typhoid

It must be remembered that these conditions above are worst case scenarios, and should be considered in conjunction with other lesions before a decision is taken.

If the enteritis is associated with emaciation the carcase and offal should be considered unfit for human consumption.

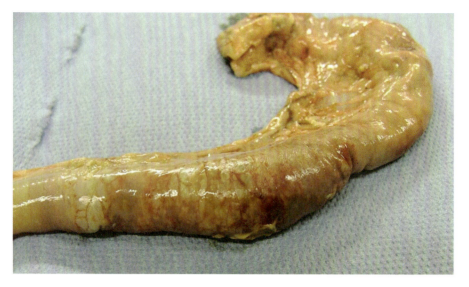

Necrotic enteritis

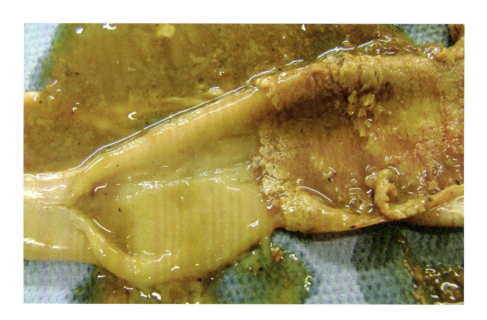

Necrotic Enteritis – Opened intestine. Note diphtheric area of necrotic mucosa and demarcation between normal and affected mucosa

FATTY LIVER SYNDROME

Livers can become enlarged, soft and friable due to the deposition of fat. In poultry, unlike mammals, almost the entire synthesis of fatty acids occurs within the liver. Causes include hormonal triggers in laying fowl, lack of exercise and high protein diets. Consequently this condition affects females; male birds affected with similar hepatic characteristics must raise suspicion of toxaemia. The liver should be rejected as unfit for human consumption.

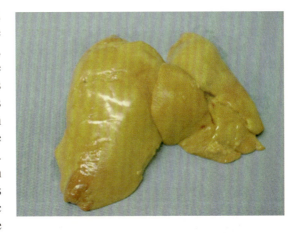

FEMORAL HEAD NECROSIS

This condition is commonly a result of blood borne bacterial infection and is classed as an osteomyelitis which can be produced by pathogens such as *Staphylococcus aureus* and *E.coli*. Although not specifically checked for during the post-mortem inspection of poultry, its' presence can be used as an indicator of bacterial infection when questions arise as to whether a septicaemic carcase is merely dehydrated or in fact diseased.

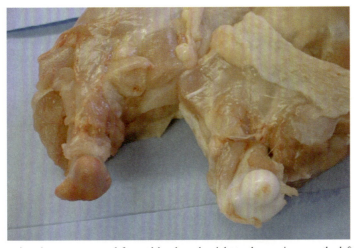

A comparison between a normal femoral head on the right to the specimen on the left from a septicaemic carcase. Note the darker thigh meat and the femoral head, which was porous and could be chipped off using fingernails.

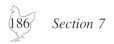

FOCAL HEPATIC NECROSIS

A condition also termed hepatic granulomas, bacterial necrosis and erroneously *E.coli*. Focal hepatic necrosis describes pinpoint whitish areas of necrosis on the liver surface and throughout the liver parenchyma. Although *E.coli* has been isolated in some cases, other bacterial strains such as *Staphylococcus aureus, Clostridium perfringens* and streptococci have also been implicated in the production of similar lesions, as have certain toxins. Judgement on the fitness for human consumption is dependant on the state of the carcase and signs of systemic spread, the liver must be rejected. If associated with pericarditis or perihepatitis the entire carcase and offal should be rejected.

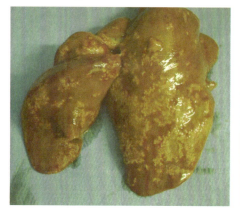

Focal hepatic necrosis – broiler

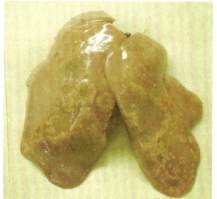

Focal hepatic necrosis – broiler. Lesion pattern typical of *Cl.perfringens* infection

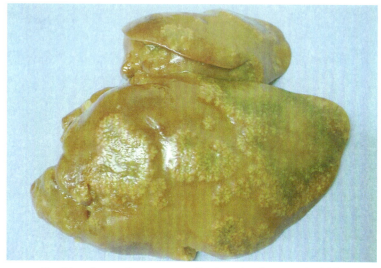

Focal hepatic granulomas – green discolouration due to retained bile

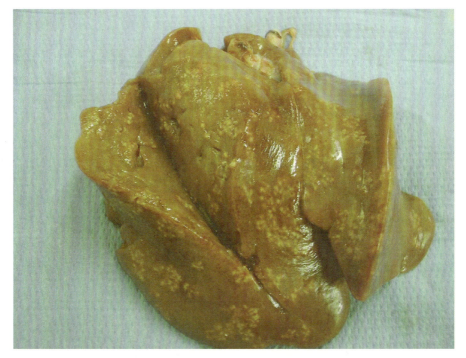

Incision into liver substance to expose granulomas.

HAEMATOPOIETIC FOCI

Haematopoietic foci are commonly found in the duodenum of broilers and should not be confused with lesions of coccidial infection, inflammation or haemorrhaging associated with the death of the animal. These areas represent an extramedullary haematopoesis (the formation of blood cells outside of the bone marrow) and are naturally occurring phenomena. The carcase and offal are fit.

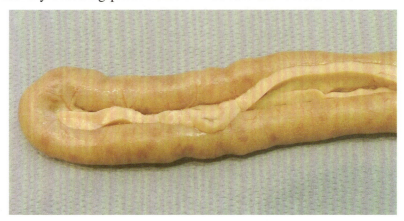

Haematopoietic foci in the duodenum

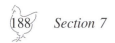

HEPATITIS

A liver fibrosis, several causes have been identified ranging from bacterial infection ascending from the intestine such as *Clostridium perfringens*, to toxins. Damage, inflammation and subsequent necrosis of the biliary system disrupt the normal flow of bile, which leaches back into the liver substance. The liver can be enlarged with a firm, smooth surface. Greenish discolouration of the liver has been noted, and the gall bladder can become thickened and distended. This condition can lead to icterus in the carcase.

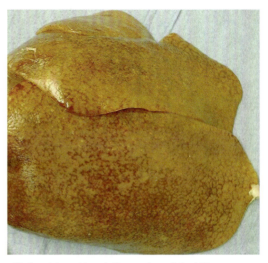

Cholangiohepatitis – inflammation of the biliary system and periportal parenchyma

Affected livers should be rejected, the carcase should be judged on its state and signs of systemic disturbance associated with hepatic disruption.

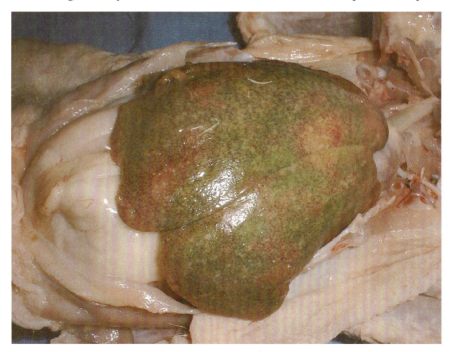

Cholangiohepatitis and reabsorbtion of bile

JAUNDICE

Also known as icterus, this condition is evidenced by discolouration of the carcase and associated offal due to the deposition of bile pigments in the body tissues owing to increased levels of bilirubin in the blood (hyperbilirubinaemia). Jaundice occurs less frequently in avian species than in mammals due to the fact that bilirubin only forms approximately 6% of bile in birds. There are two main forms of icterus, hepatic or obstructive. In hepatic icterus the cause is disruption of hepatic cells through disease or poisoning. Obstructive icterus occurs when the flow of bile into the duodenum is disrupted by factors such as enteritis or cholangitis (inflammation of the bile ducts) and a failure to remove bile pigments from the intestine by absorption through the intestinal mucosa and returning them to the liver via the portal circulation. In poultry this condition is usually due to hepatic disease.

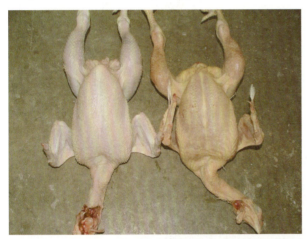

A jaundiced bird on the right compared with a normal bird on left.

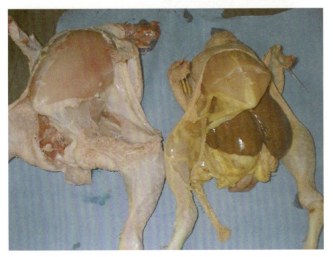

The same two carcases with ribcage and skin reflected. Note enlarged liver, yellowish tinge of tissues and fat.

Clinical signs vary with the nature of the cause of the hepatic disturbance. Unfeathered areas of skin appear yellow; in severe cases the eyes are coloured, as are the mucous membranes of the mouth. Tissues and organs of the body will be pigmented yellow; the liver is normally enlarged and yellow tinged.

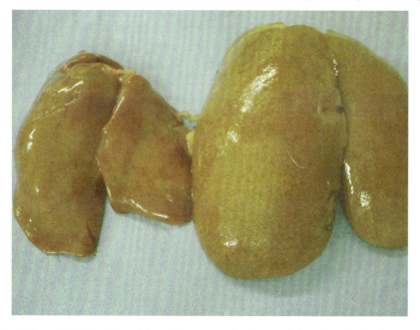

Enlarged liver with cholangiohepatitis on right compared with normal liver from similar sized bird. In this case the carcase was rejected for hepatic jaundice.

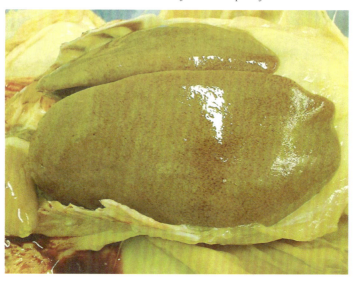

A second example of cholangiohepatitis as a finding in a case of jaundice in a broiler.

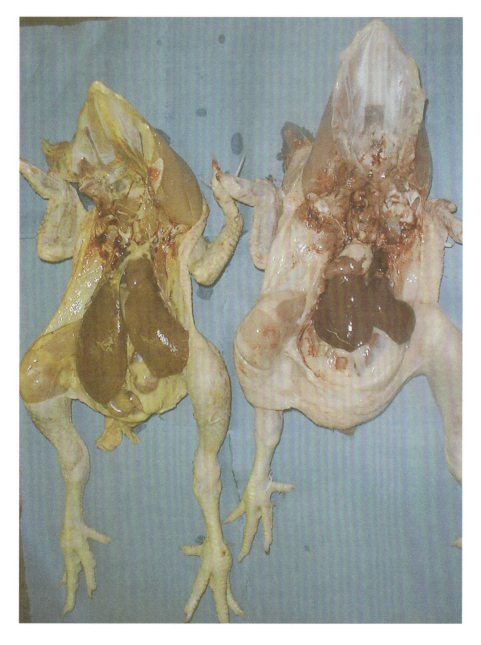

Jaundice due to hepatitis affecting carcase on left

Carcase and offal are unfit for human consumption.

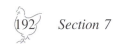

PENDULOUS CROP

An enlarged crop containing foul-smelling contents caused by factors such as paralysis of nerves, excessive water consumption or partial blockage of the alimentary tract due to food impaction. Fungal organisms can further infect the contents. If associated with emaciation, septicaemia or abnormal odour the carcase should be rejected as unfit for human consumption. If detected at the whole bird inspection point the risk of contamination of machinery, and hence further carcases if the crop is ruptured, must be taken into consideration.

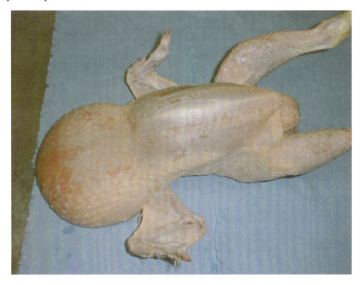

Pendulous crop in a broiler

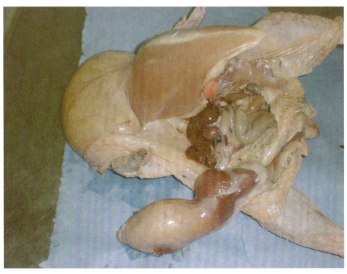

Partial dissection showing impacted proventriculus.

PERICARDITIS

Pericarditis is the inflammation of the serous sac surrounding the heart known as the pericardium. Pericarditis can take many forms, from a cloudy formation on the otherwise transparent membrane, through to adhesion between the epicardium and the pericardium, to complete fibrinous, purulent pericarditis.

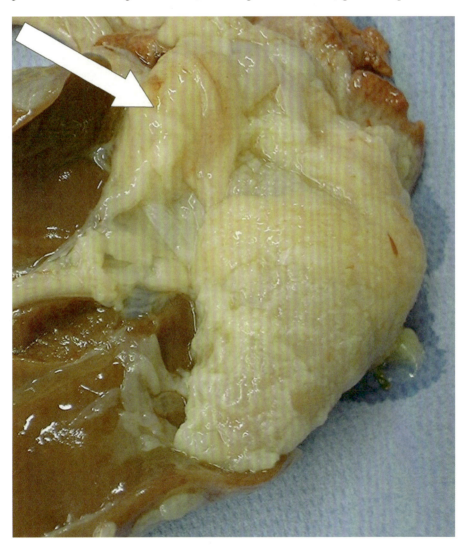

Purulent Epicarditis and pericarditis (Pericardium removed and arrowed)

Most serotypes of *E.coli* will produce pericarditis, and a more fluid pericarditis is an indicator of a septicaemic condition, including that due to *Salmonella enteriditis* which is often associated with a mucopurulent exudate within a distended pericardium. Adhesion of the pericardium to the surface of the heart can also be due to conditions such as Campylobacterosis.

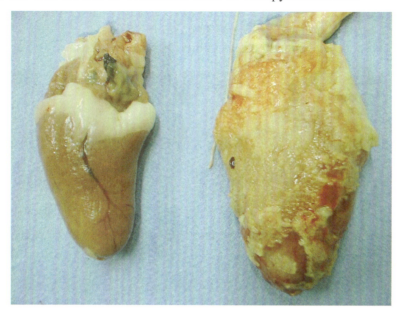

Purulent Epicarditis of heart on right compared to normal on left

Carcases and offal presenting with pericarditis are rejected as unfit for human consumption due to the high incidence of pericarditis caused by pathogenic bacteria transmissible to humans.

PERITONITIS / PERIHEPATITIS

Peritonitis is a term describing inflammation of the peritoneum, a membrane that lines the walls of the abdominal cavity and the internal organs. The part of the membrane lining the abdominal wall is termed the parietal membrane, the section covering the internal organs is known as the visceral peritoneum. The peritoneum is a serous membrane, it secretes a watery fluid that provides nutrients and lubricates.

Egg peritonitis is an infection of laying fowl due to bacterial infection of yolk material that is released into the abdominal cavity. This release and subsequent infection can be triggered by, for example, ovarian regression, a rising oviduct infection, or ovarian rupture. Egg peritonitis is usually characterised by a yellow, cheesy exudate covering the abdominal cavity and the viscera, this exudate is normally associated with a foul odour and should not be confused with lesions associated with conditions such as airsacculitis.

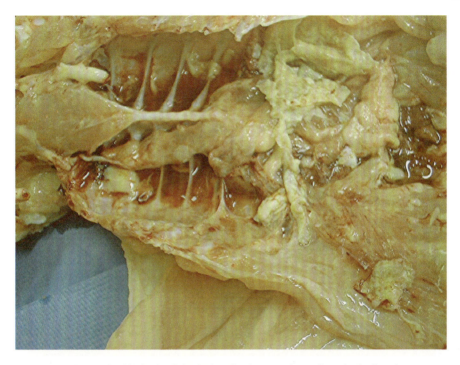

Purulent peritonitis in the abdominal cavity from a primary focus in the intestines

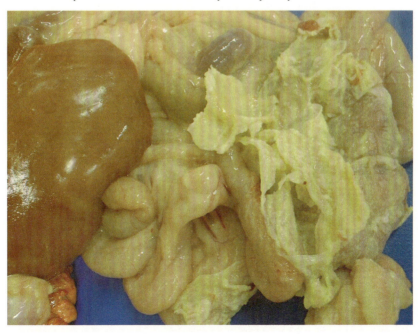

Visceral peritonitis. Pus adherent to the small intestine at the point of the diverticulum suggests an initial yolk sac infection as the primary foci

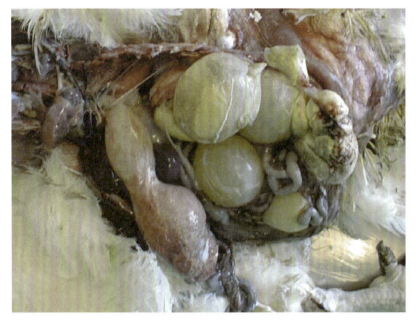

Visceral peritonitis – ovaries, proventriculus and gizzard, commercial layer

Perihepatitis is a specific form of visceral peritonitis affecting the peritoneum covering the liver and is principally associated with *E.coli* infection. Perihepatitis can range from areas of adherent fibrous attachment to gross thickening of the capsule, which becomes opaque.

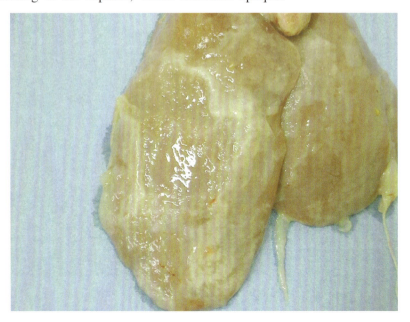

Perihepatitis – Fibrin on surface of broiler liver

Traumatic peritonitis is a specific condition where infection is caused by injury, most commonly due to a foreign object. Broilers are indiscriminate eaters, and will swallow anything they think is food. This means that occasionally nails and pieces of wire are eaten. These objects can then be forced through the walls of the gizzard due to its grinding movement and set up an infection. When an infection is created by the presence of a nail or wire, a black pus forms in the abdominal cavity, this pus also has an offensive odour. More often than not, the evisceration equipment will not remove the offal as the peritonitis glues it into the cavity.

Carcases with peritonitis or perihepatitis should be rejected as unfit for human consumption.

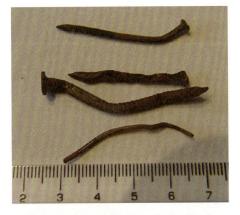

A selection of 'hardware' removed from one flock of broilers at evisceration

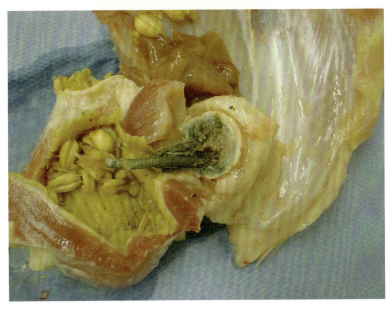

A piece of wire projecting through the gizzard and perforating the sternum

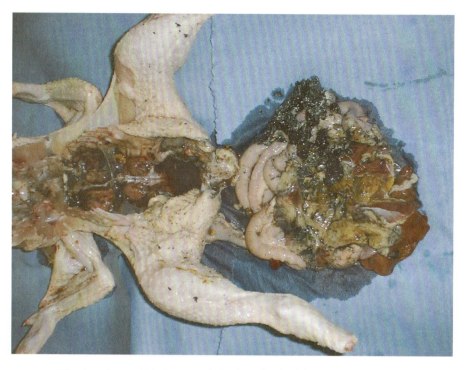

Offensive odour and black pus are indicative of peritonitis due to metallic objects

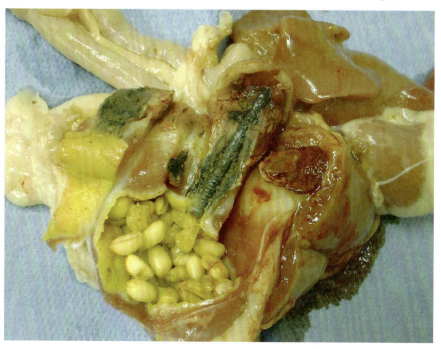

An incised gizzard, revealing a nail forced through its' walls

PODODERMATITIS

Pododermatitis is an inflammation of the plantar surface or pad of the foot. The affected area exhibits all the characteristic signs of inflammation; localized swelling, heat, pain, redness and disturbance of function. Affected birds show signs of lameness and pain. Frequently pododermatitis leads to 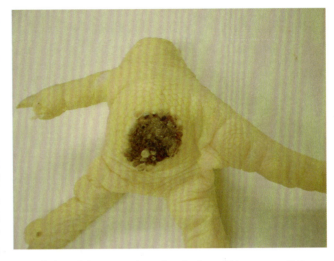 necrosis and desquamation of the skin covering the lesion. Litter conditions, especially damp areas around feeders are thought to be the main cause. Affected feet should be rejected as unfit for human consumption. The level of pododermatitis within a flock is indicative of the environmental conditions on farm and can range from a slight discolouration and hyperkeratosis (thickening) of the skin to deep ulceration, at which point it is termed plantar necrosis.

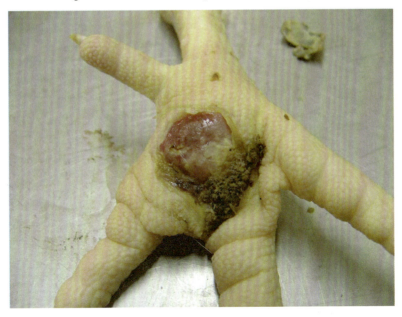

Severe pododermatitis

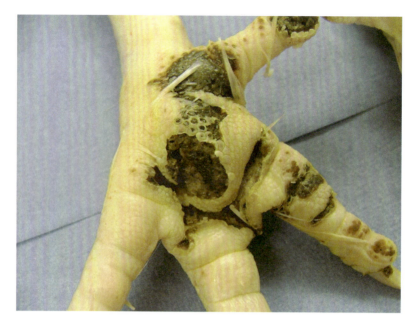

Deep ulceration associated with plantar necrosis

RUPTURED GASTROCNEMIUS TENDON (GREEN LEG DISEASE)

Green leg disease is a condition where bruising occurs in the legs due to the tendon at the rear of the hock snapping, it can be uni or bi-lateral. It appears as a green discolouration of the leg and the ruptured tendon can be felt by pushing at the area of muscle near the hock joint. The aetiology of the lesion ranges from the infectious, such as viral or bacterial tenosynovitis, to non-infectious causes. Affected parts should be rejected.

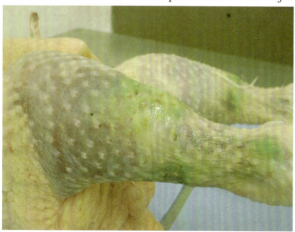

Greenish discolouration of the legs

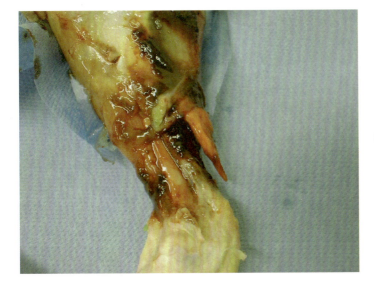

Skin removed to reveal
ruptured tendon

SALPINGITIS

This term describes inflammation of the salpinx, the oviduct. There are many causes of this inflammatory response including an *E.coli* infection rising from the vagina, *Mycoplasma spp* infection, Infectious Bronchitis, viral infection and transfer of infection from the abdominal airsacs. In the latter case the salpingitis is viewed as being part of an airsacculitis complex. Salpingitis is particularly common in ducks, especially as a lesion associated with anatipestifer infection.

Salpingitis can lead to egg peritonitis in laying fowl due to the inability of released ova to enter the occluded oviduct, they then become prone to bacterial infection when present in the abdominal cavity. The infected oviduct can become grossly enlarged, and may be impacted with a cheese-like core. If the lesion is localised with no evidence of systemic involvement the affected area should be trimmed and rejected.

If the salpingitis is associated with abnormal odour, septicaemia, emaciation , or other sign of systemic, spread the entire carcase and associated offal should be considered unfit for human consumption.

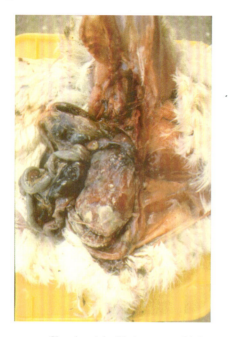

Chronic salpingitis in a young bird

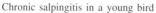

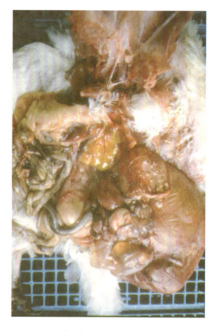

Salpingitis in a mature bird

SEPTICAEMIA / TOXAEMIA

Septicaemia, toxaemia and pyrexia (fever) are umbrella terms that describe a group of lesions encountered at inspection, as in general, it is not possible to diagnose causative organisms on the line.

Septicaemia – This condition denotes systemic disease caused by bacteria multiplying in the bloodstream. The characteristic lesions are due to a combination of increased body temperature (hyperthermia) including dehydration and loss of skin elasticity. The meat is soft and dark and can be clearly seen at the whole bird inspection point. The liver generally has a 'par-boiled' appearance (cloudy swelling) due to cellular expansion and small haemorrhages (petechiae) are normally evident in the serous membranes of the liver, heart and lungs.

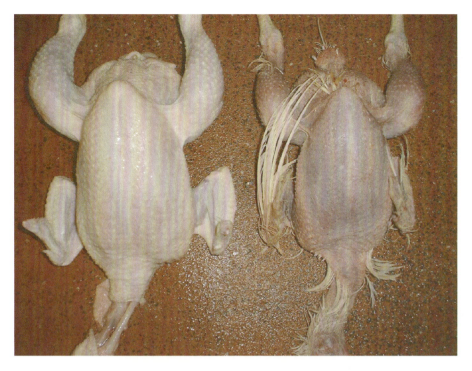

A septicaemic carcase on the right compared to unaffected carcase

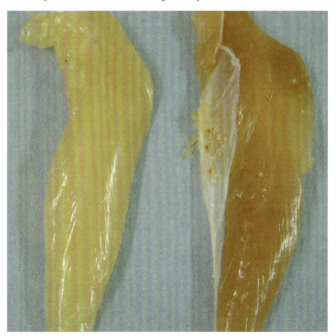

Darker supracoracoideus muscle from a septicaemic carcase on right

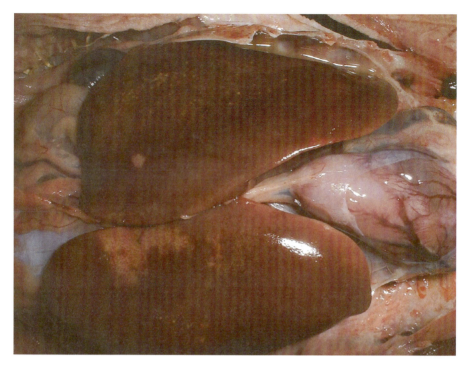

Hepatic lesions, cloudy swelling of heart. Note prominent blood vessels on heart

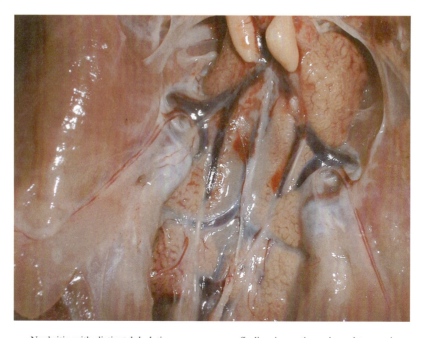

Nephritis with distinct lobulations – a common finding in septicaemia and toxaemia

Toxaemia, is the presence of toxins, normally bacterial in origin, in the bloodstream. Certain bacteria including *Clostridium spp* possess the ability to increase their invasive potential by producing protein exotoxins, others, especially coliforms, produce endotoxins from their lipopolysaccharide cell walls when they break down. Large quantities of toxin in the blood leads to a condition known as toxic shock, manifested by abnormally high heart rate (tachycardia) and dilation of peripheral blood vessels, which may rupture. Petechial haemorrhaging of soft tissues including heart, lungs and skin is a common finding.

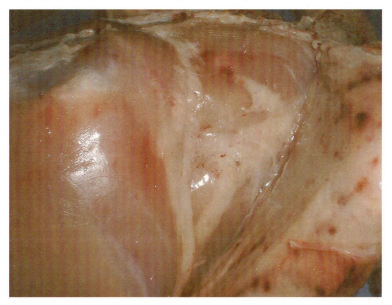

Petechial haemorrhaging of the skin (reflected) and subcutaneous musculature

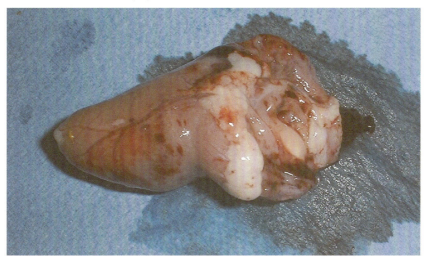

Cardiac petechiae

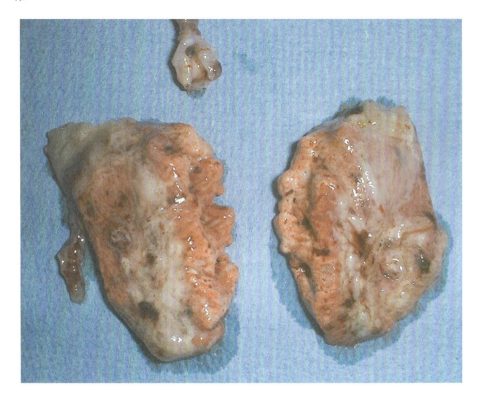

Ruptured blood vessels in lung tissue

Pyrexia – Fever, elevated body temperature in response to an infective agent, and forms part of the body's immune response. The respiration and pulse rate increases and leads to a fevered carcase being darker as the surface blood vessels become dilated and contain more blood. Internal organs undergo a cloudy swelling which, if the condition is chronic, may lead to the deposition of fat in damaged cells (fatty degeneration.)

Colibacillosis – infection by *Escherichia coli* can be septicaemic or toxaemic. *E.coli* tends to be a secondary invader, initial weakening of the immune system due to *Mycoplasma spp.* infections for example, allow *E.coli* to spread. The carcase displays the lesions associated with septicaemia, the offal presents with characteristic lesions of fibrinous polyserositis which can become inspissated especially over the liver.

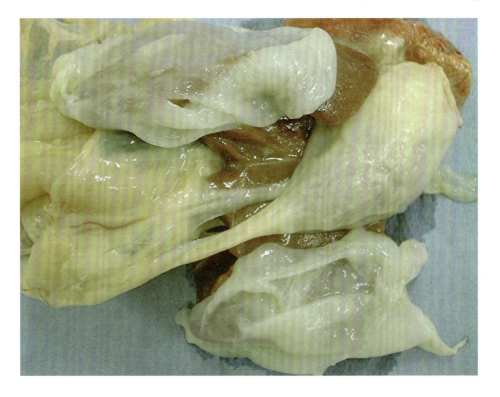

The fibrinous perihepatitis and pericarditis associated with colibacillosis.

Coligranuloma – Hjärre's Disease, an *E.coli* infection characterised by granulomas in the intestinal wall, liver and lungs. This tends to be a chronic condition and more likely to be found in layers and spent hens than in broiler age birds. The granulomas, when incised, possess layered pus atypical of *E.coli* infections, which can be used as a diagnositic aid in differentiating this condition from similar lesions associated with adenocarcinomas which are smooth and glossy when incised.

Septicaemia, toxaemia and pyrexia all produce similar characteristics in the carcase. Due to dehydration the skin loses elasticity, a test employed at the inspection point being to pinch the skin, which will normally spring back in a healthy bird, but will remain out in unhealthy birds.

Carcases displaying lesions consistent with these conditions are considered unfit for human consumption and should be rejected with their associated offal.

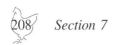

SKIN LESIONS

Breast Blisters – These are due to distension of the sternal bursa with fluid either through trauma or pressure. This blister tends to occur in heavier birds such as turkeys that become recumbent and spend time supporting their weight on the keel, and in poultry housed in systems with percheries. These blisters can be prone to secondary infection, setting up a septicaemia within the carcase. Infected blisters with no signs of systemic spread may be trimmed. If the affected tissue is adherent to the sternum, part of the bone should be removed with the affected tissue. Small, non-haemorrhagic blisters may be deferred until after the chilling process, when a proportion of them will have disappeared.

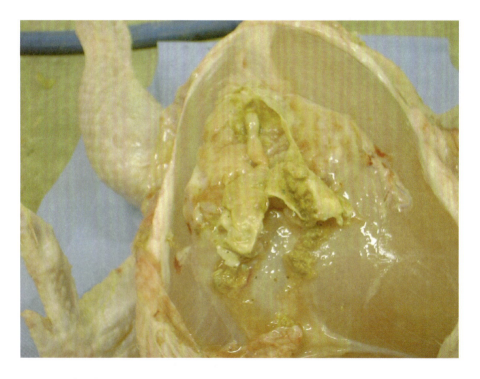

Infected sternal bursa. Skin reflected to show cellulitis and adherence to sternum

Cellulitis – This is inflammation between the skin and muscle caused by infection of the connective tissue. It can occur in any area of the body but the most common form encountered is pericloacal cellulitis around the vent area and upper thighs in broilers. At the wholebird inspection point the condition presents as a yellowing and thickening (hyperkeratosis) of the skin which when incised reveals the seropurulent lesion beneath. There are two forms of cellulitis, wet and dry. In the wet form the connective tissue below the skin is yellowish and jellylike, with areas of yellow caseous pus, the wet form is frequently associated with septicaemia. The dry form, known as 'crisping' consists of a sheet of dry, inspissated pus, under which the tissue surface frequently displays redness due to dilation of capillaries as part of the immune response.

It has been my experience that poor feathering, and conditions in a broiler shed that promote pododermatitis, appears to increase the incidence of cellulitis within the flock. The area above the lesion tends to be frequently associated with scratch scarring suggesting that the inoculation of environmental contaminants may be the major source of this condition. *E.coli* has been the causative organism most frequently isolated from active lesions and as such carcases with cellulitis are rejected as unfit for human consumption.

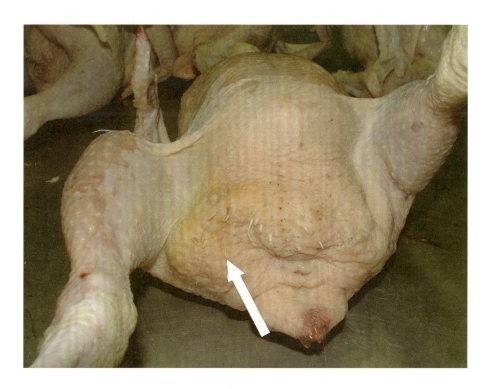

Pericloacal cellulitis – yellowing and hyperkeratosis. This can be bilateral

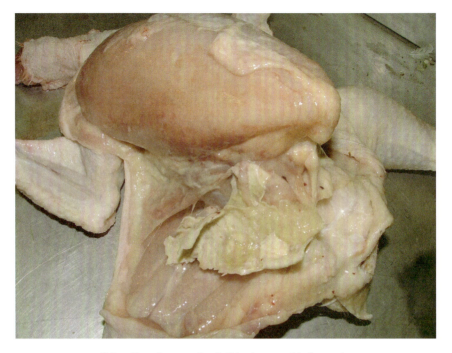

Skin reflected to reveal cellulitis plaque and inflammation

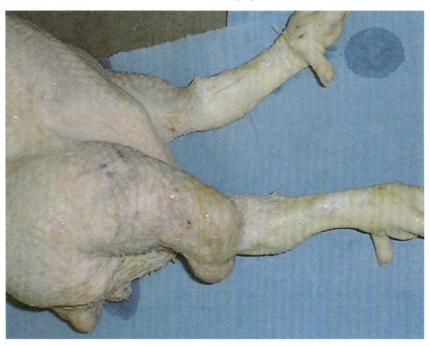

Cellulitis lesions in the hock area

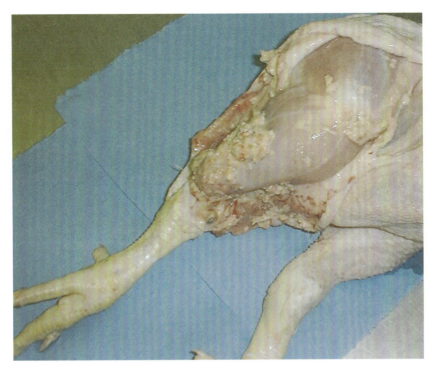

Skin reflected – possibly a secondary bacterial infection following tenosynovitis

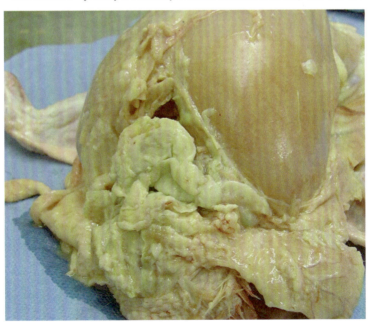

An infected thoracic inlet in a broiler

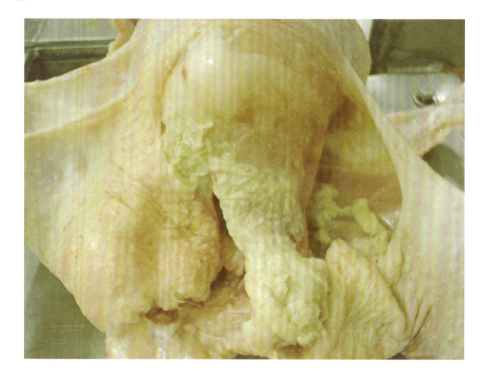

The wet form of cellulitis, this becomes inspissated and develops into the parchment-like lesion associated with the dry form

DERMATITIS

Inflammation of the skin. This can be due to contact irritation with wet litter, (when it appears most frequently on the sternum), nutritional deficiencies, trauma and bacterial infection.

BREAST BURN

A contact / pressure necrosis of the skin overlying the sternum following prolonged contact with an irritant, usually wet litter. A high percentage of lesions within a flock can be considered an indication of the environmental conditions during the rearing period. The affected part can be trimmed and rejected, however an examination for secondary bacterial infection such as cellulitis should be carried out.

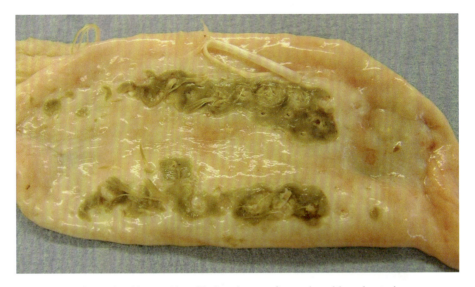

A sample of breast skin – blackened areas of necrosis and hyperkeratosis

SCABBY HIP DERMATITIS

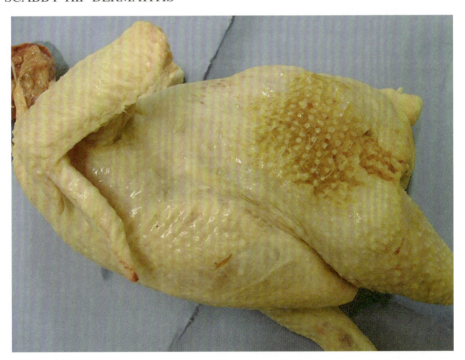

Scabby hip dermatitis

Thought to be partly due to biotin deficiency and the prevalence of scratches, this condition presents as a discolouration of the hip area due to the accumulation of necrotic debris on the surface. Generally the feather follicles themselves are uninfected and can be seen through the 'scab'. The carcase is considered fit for human consumption after removal of the affected skin, however if there are indications of cellulitis under the lesions the carcase should be rejected.

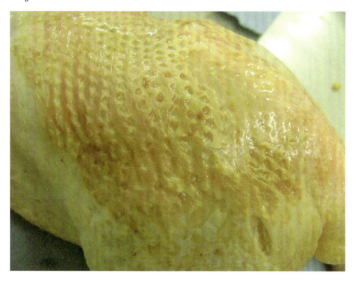

Scabby hip dermatitis – lesions extending across the back

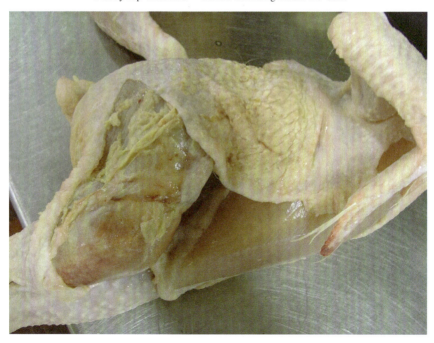

Cellulitis associated with scabby hip dermatitis, note thickened skin

Gangrenous Dermatitis - Also known as Necrotic Dermatitis, Gangrenous cellulitis, Avian Malignant Oedema. Localised wounds in the skin lead to bacterial invasion. Several *Clostridial* spp of bacteria are associated with this condition with *Cl.septicum* being most prevalent. Certain disease complexes such as those leading to anaemia appear to reduce immunity to gangrenous dermatitis that mostly affects the skin of the legs and abdomen.

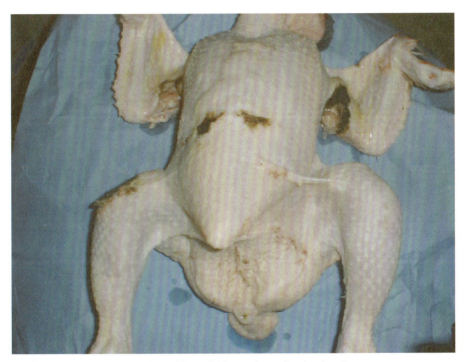

Necrotic dermatitis on the breast, leg and under the wings

Gross Lesions include necrosis of the skin, subcutaneous fluid, muscle with cooked appearance and haemorrhaging.

Gas may also be produced under the skin and in the muscle tissue, producing a dry, crackling sound (crepitation) when the affected tissue is pressed.

Carcase and offal are unfit for human consumption.

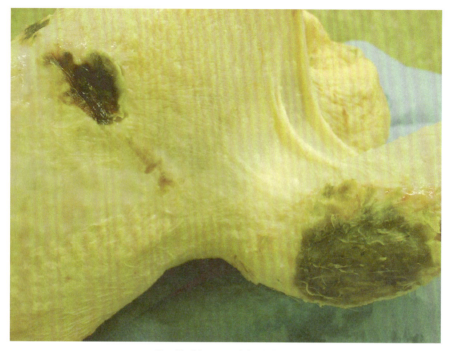

Detail of breast and leg lesions

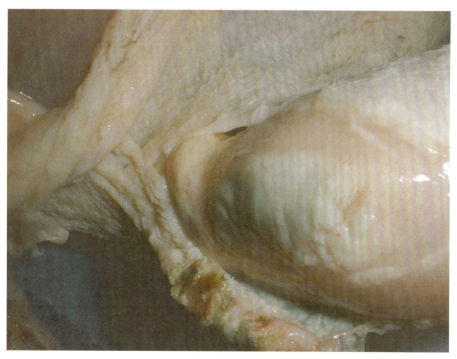

Detail of leg lesion – skin reflected

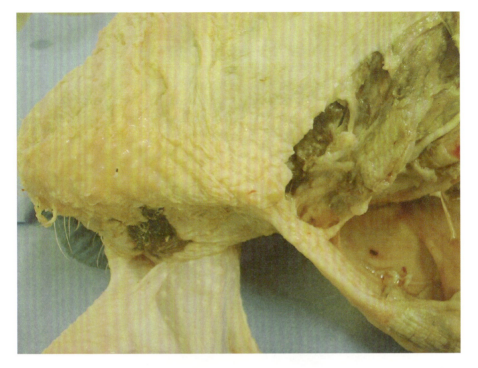

Extensive gangrenous lesions visible through the skin

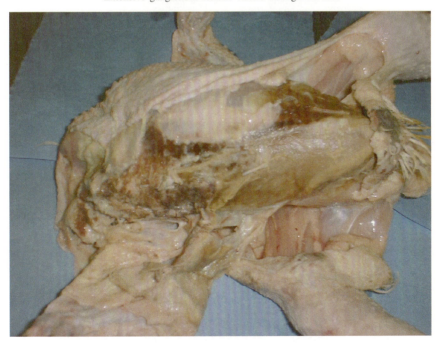

Skin reflected revealing extensive areas of necrosis

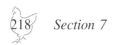

CHRONIC BACTERIAL DERMATITIS

Chronic bacterial dermatitis presents as a hyperkeratosis of the skin and is usually associated with cyanosis of the carcase. In the live bird sparse feather cover, possibly due to factors such as amino acid deficiency, can lead to bacterial colonisation of feather follicles. Inoculation through scratches of skin unprotected by feathers may also introduce infection. If associated with cyanosis, septicaemia or cellulitis the carcase is unfit for human consumption.

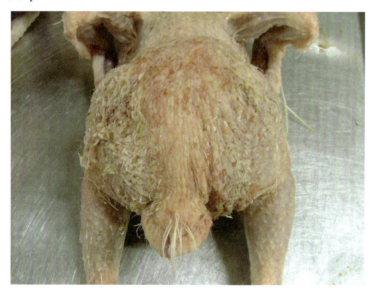

Chronic bacterial dermatitis

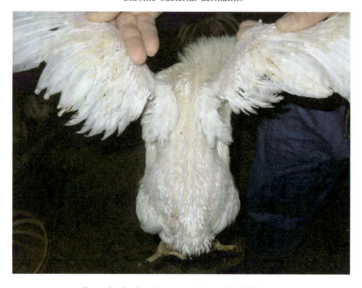

Poor feathering due to amino acid deficiency

FOLLICULITIS

Inflammation of the feather follicles can occur due to various reasons including bacterial colonisation and viruses such as Marek's disease. The photographs following illustrate acute folliculitis of the inner thighs presented in 34% of a single flock slaughtered during the summer.

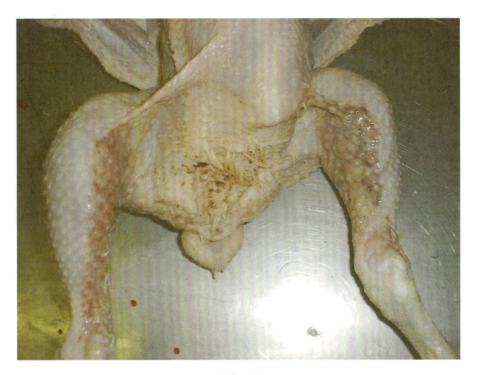

Folliculitis

The lesions were pustular, foul smelling and were associated with high rejection rates for dehydration/cyanosis, cellulitis and dermatitis. On investigation it transpired that large numbers of birds had died in the shed partly due to abnormally hot and humid environmental conditions and the affected birds had been literally 'straddling' the corpses.

If folliculitis is associated with other lesions characterising Marek's disease the carcase and offal are unfit. It is also unfit if presenting with cyanosis, septicaemia, cellulitis or abnormal odour.

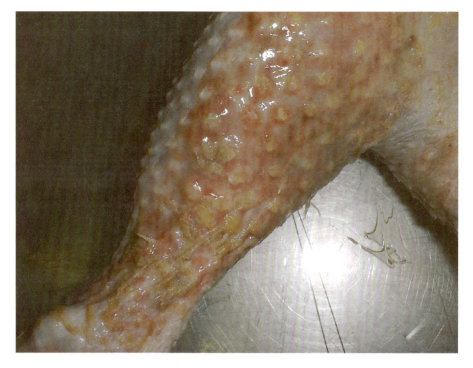

Folliculitis – detail of pustular feather follicles and Cutaneous inflammatory response

HOCKBURN

The term hockburn is a misnomer; the lesions are a contact/pressure necrosis of the dermis covering the hocks of similar multifactorial aetiology to pododermatitis. Before the removal of mammalian protein from poultry feed this lesions was considered to ostensibly be due to contact with acid high nitrogen content faeces, literally a burn. Since the removal of this feed constituent the prevalence of this lesion has diminished, however it still exists. Anecdotal evidence suggests that although the environmental conditions during the rearing period can cause or exacerbate both pododermatitis and hockburn, the lesions do not always manifest themselves at the same time. Damage to the integrity of the dermis can lead to secondary bacterial infection and conditions such as tenosynovitis, but if uncomplicated the bird is fit for consumption. Owing to the public perception of hockburn, most processors will attempt to remove it and most retailers will not accept it for wholebirds. A high incidence of hockburn within a flock should be considered as an indication of poor welfare conditions on farm.

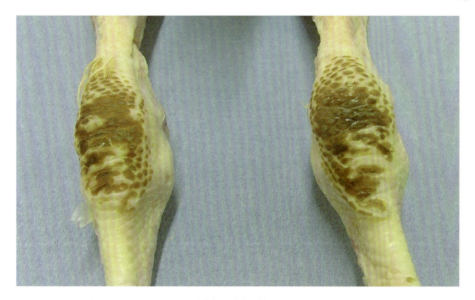

Bi-lateral hockburn

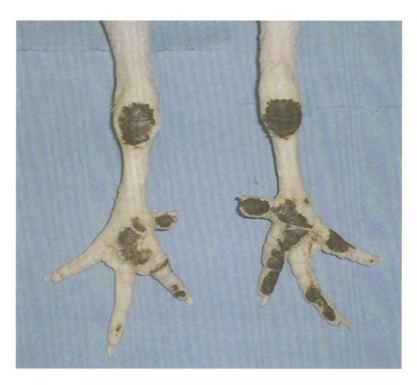

Bi-lateral hockburn and pododermatitis

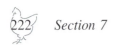

CONGENITAL DEFORMITIES

These present as variation from the norm. If the bird and carcase show no ill effects of this variation they are considered fit for human consumption. In some cases rejection of the affected part may be warranted if the deformity would be considered aesthetically repugnant by the final consumer or would pose a contamination risk in automated evisceration lines. The commonest lesions encountered include:

Polydactylia – Extra digits or limbs. The appearance of additional non-functional limbs does occur in poultry. Removal of the limb is usually all that is required however if this is not possible and the location of the limb could cause evisceration problems it poses a contamination risk and the carcase should be rejected.

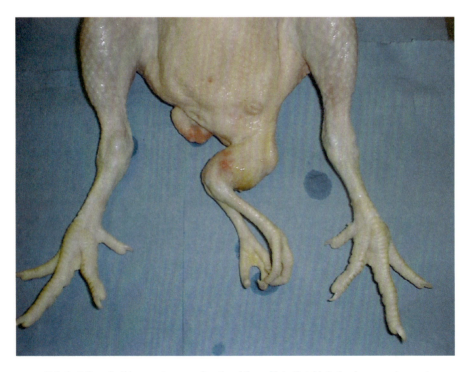

Polydactylia – in this case two non-functional legs. Note that bird also has an extra vent

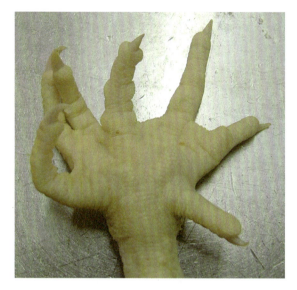

A seven toed foot – A congenital defect that did not affect the growth of the bird

Persistent Right Oviduct – Regression of the right oviduct occurs early in the life of a female chicken, with only the left ovary and oviduct developing to maturity. Occasionally the occluded remnant of the right oviduct fills with fluid derived from the blood plasma and forms a clear cyst attached to the cloaca. The carcase and offal are fit for human consumption.

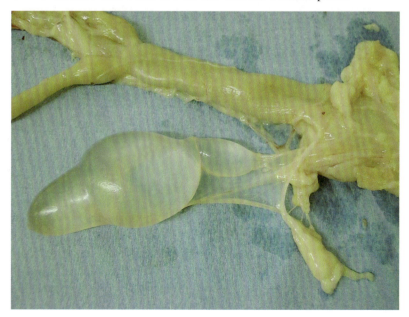

Cystic right oviduct

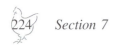

STERNAL ABNORMALITIES

Sternal abnormalities are an incidental finding and usually take the form of failure in the development of the posterior keel bone of the sternum. There is a small risk of possible carcase contamination during automated evisceration processes. In the live bird, hepatic trauma can occur owing to the loss of skeletal protection for the posterior parietal surface of the liver. The carcase and associated offal are fit for human consumption, although processors may elect to portion the carcase for aesthetic reasons.

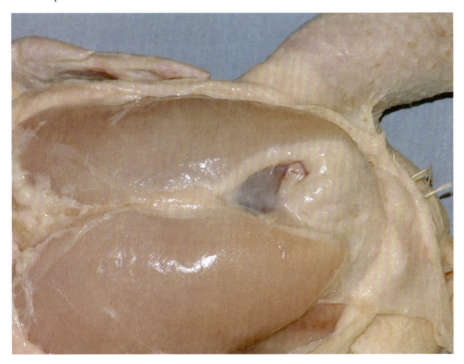

Sternal abnormality – skin refelected. Note proximity of liver to surface.

DIGESTIVE ABNORMALITIES

These include conditions such as extraneous caeca and occlusions of the digestive tract. The presence of extra functional/non-functional digestive tract parts does not normally affect the fitness of the carcase. Occlusions of the digestive tract tend to increase in size and become filled with partially digested, usually fermenting material and gas. As such they present a serious contamination risk during hand or automated evisceration and should be considered for rejection. In general, occlusions of parts of the digestive tract also affect the function of this system which will be evident in the entire carcase as emaciation. It may be possible, for example with large turkey carcases that show no signs of emaciation or systemic disturbance, to salvage the carcase if the evisceration can be carried out with special precautions to prevent rupture of the intestinal lesion.

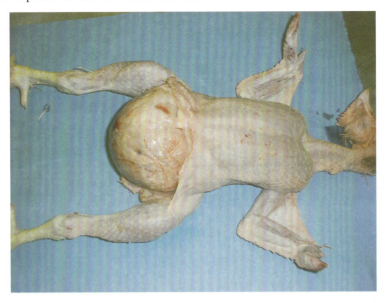

Occlusion of the ileum – formation of a distended intestine preventing evisceration

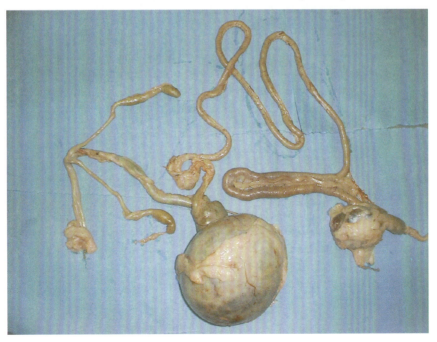

Removed intestinal tract – Cyanosis of the carcase and enteritis warranted rejection of the carcase

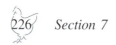

CARDIAC ABNORMALITIES

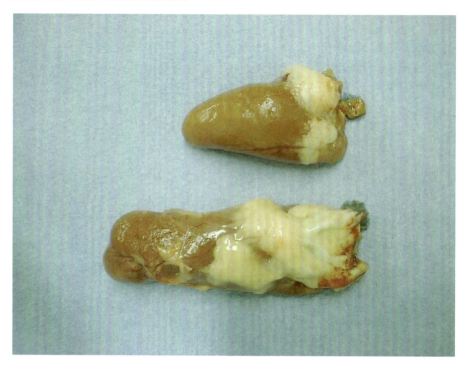

Congenital cardiac anomaly of lower heart compared with normal above

As with other congenital abnormalities, cardiac lesions such as that pictured above are an incidental finding at post mortem inspection. If the abnormality has had no detrimental affect on the growth of the bird the carcase and offal are fit for human consumption

BRACHIAL CYSTS

These present as fluid filled cysts attached to the proventriculus. They are of rare occurrence but can affect the normal function of the proventriculus and hence the digestive processes of the bird, in addition to applying physical pressure on other organs in the vicinity.

The carcase and offal are fit for consumption unless there are signs of emaciation due to disturbance of the digestive system in which case total rejection is warranted.

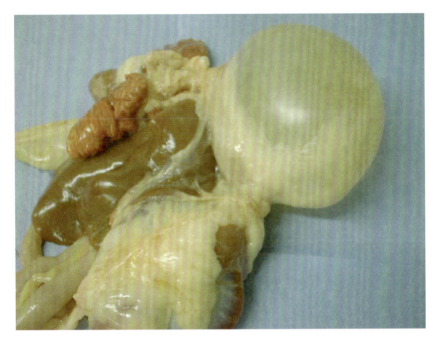

A large brachial cyst attached to the proventriculus

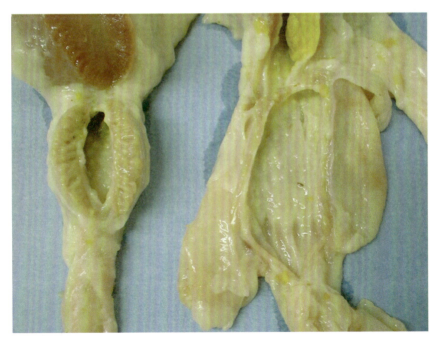

Incision of the affected proventriculus illustrating atrophy of the glandular cells and damage to the internal mucosa. Healthy proventriculus on left for comparison. Carcase was rejected for emaciation.

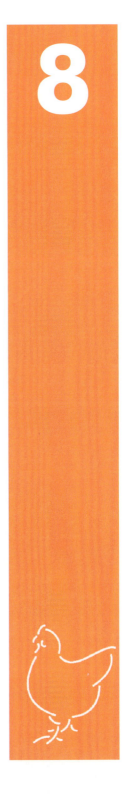

PROCESSING CONDITIONS

8

CONTAMINATION

Poultry meat, carcases and/or offal affected with gross contamination by faecal material, bile, grease, disinfectants etc should be considered unfit for human consumption.

INTESTINAL CONTAMINATION

Contamination due to rupture of pendulous crops. Either reject carcase before evisceration, or, if the carcase is in good condition, detain the carcase and trim out the crop before evisceration. Contamination occurring at the vent cut or neck area should be removed by trimming the affected area. Contamination of the skin may be washed off if undertaken immediately using a low-pressure spray and copious quantity of water. Slight to moderate cavity contamination may be washed out by placing the carcase vertically over a spray to facilitate drainage.

Gross contamination renders the carcase and offal unfit for human consumption. It may be possible to salvage some cuts provided this may be achieved hygienically. Contaminated offal is unfit for human consumption.

BILE STAINING

Parts affected by bile staining should be trimmed and rejected as unfit for human consumption.

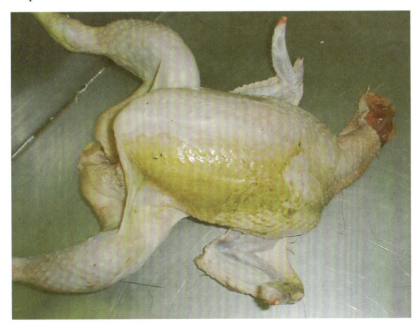

Bile from a gall bladder ruptured during evisceration evident on a broiler carcase

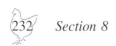

POULTRY MEAT FALLING FROM THE LINE, CONVEYOR ETC

Offal falling on the floor or other contaminated surface, carcases or offal falling into feather flumes or evisceration troughs, and portions of deboned poultry meat falling onto the floor or other potentially contaminated surface should be considered unfit. Carcases falling onto the floor or other potentially contaminated surface may be picked up and immediately washed if the floor or surface appears clean and the carcase is picked up within a few minutes of falling and exposed muscle is trimmed under supervision.

DEATH OTHER THAN SLAUGHTER

As slaughter is defined as 'death by exsanguination', death other than slaughter simply implies that the bird was not bled. This can be due to several causes, the most obvious being that the bird missed the automatic cutters (if they are used) and was subsequently missed by the back-up slaughter person. Or if a manual system is used, that the slaughter person either missed the bird or failed to cut the bird properly. As such, the monitoring of the rate of uncut birds is vitally important as it is of welfare concern particularly when high frequency stunning systems are used (and birds are not killed in the stunning process), and any occurrence should be investigated.

The neck cut will be absent or will be found to be insufficient to have caused death by loss of blood. In addition to being darker skinned than normal due to the presence of blood in the sub dermal area, birds suspended upside down will display swollen, enlarged blood engorged heads and blood coloured necks.

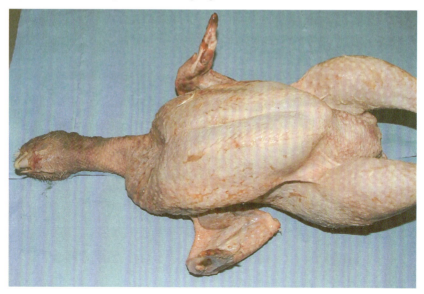

An 'uncut' broiler. Note the swelling of the head

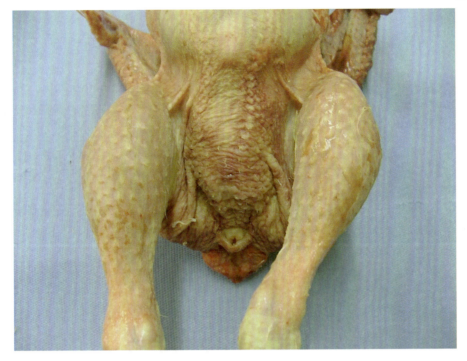

Congestion of the skin and pygostyle

Birds that have died due to causes other than slaughter are to be rejected as unfit for human consumption.

DEAD ON ARRIVAL

Through the stresses imposed on the birds during catching, transportation, lairaging and even illness, the finding of dead birds at the point of hanging on is unfortunately a common occurrence. Obviously, in terms of bird welfare, death during this period represents the ultimate welfare insult and as such should be carefully monitored to ascertain any underlying trends such as farm, catching team, time of day of depopulation, ambient temperature, length of journey, haulier, route of journey and length of time between arrival and processing. It is important to remember that any increase in the number of birds found dead also indicates that the welfare of the flock or load as a whole has been compromised.

The cause of death in these cases range from the traumatic, such as the dislocation of the femur and subsequent haemorrhage, to heat stress and suffocation.

On conducting a post mortem examination lividity is generally found, denoting gravitational drainage of the blood to the lower points of the body.

Cyanosis of skeletal muscles is common, especially in cases where death occurred due to heat stress, anoxia and asphyxia; due to increased levels of myoglobin. Opening the carcase should give an indication of the cause of death especially if due to disease, conditions such as ascites, or trauma such as hepatic rupture. Congestion of the internal organs is common.

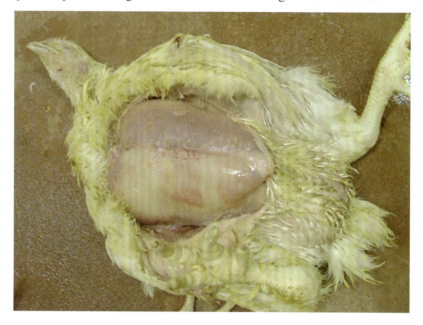

Lividity of the left breast evident on this 'found dead' bird

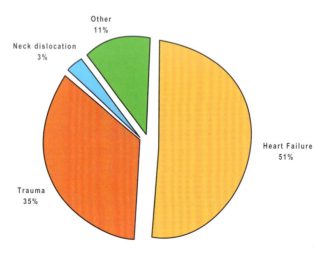

Causes of 'Found dead' in a survey.   Source: AW Training, DFAS Langford

Birds that are found dead must not be processed and should be rejected as unfit for human consumption.

MACHINE DAMAGE

Breaks in the skin can occur during the plucking process, the assessment of the fitness of the carcase should centre on the state of the subcutaneous tissue and musculature, in terms of damage and possible contamination risks. Localised trimming may suffice in most cases, however deep tissue damage should result in rejection of the affected part.

Carcases extensively damaged or mutilated by machinery should be rejected as unfit for human consumption.

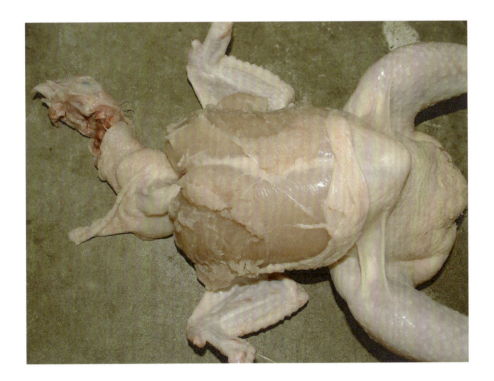

Mutilation of the breast in this broiler carcase caused by the rubber fingers of the plucking machine

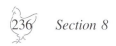

OVERSCALD

Overscalding of poultry carcases is a rejection condition due to a failure in the processing system. The slaughter process for poultry generally involves passing the bird through a tank of heated water to open the feather follicles to facilitate subsequent ease of plucking. These tanks are held at a temperature of between 50-53°C (soft scald mainly for fresh market), or around 63°C (hard scald, mainly used for frozen market), in which the birds normally pass through within approximately 2 minutes. Any malfunction in the mechanical system, deviation in scald tank temperature, alteration of the line speed (including the line stopping) can affect the carcase. Line stoppages obviously increase the time the carcase spends in the tank, during which time the meat can literally cook.

Overscalded carcases lose their protective epidermis and become greasy to the touch and the breast muscle turns white. In cases of doubt, the breast muscle should be incised, if the white, cooked appearance is evident to a depth of greater than 2mm the carcase should be rejected.

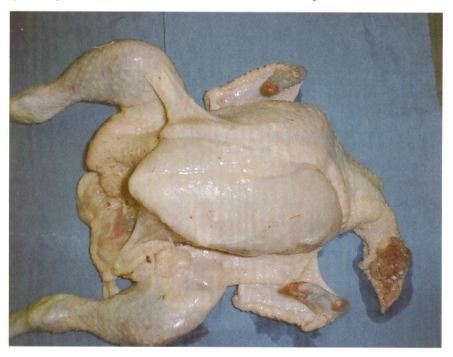

An overscalded carcase - note the waxy appearance of the skin and the cooked muscle

In the case of turkeys or larger birds, the carcases may be detained and unaffected meat may be salvaged under supervision.

THERMAL DISTRESS

In common with all living organisms, poultry have a range of temperatures, a thermal 'comfort zone,' in which they thrive. Ambient temperatures that fall outside of this range affect the internal temperature of the bird and can produce thermal distress, the severity of the bird reaction to this stress being dependent on various factors. In general poultry have a better ability to cope with temperatures below their optimum range (hypothermia) than they do with temperatures above this range (hyperthermia), the average broiler has a rectal temperature of approximately 41.5°C, with fatality occurring with an 11°C drop of body temperature or a 5°C rise. In cold conditions bird temperature is increased by shivering, increased metabolic activity and conducted heat produced by huddling together.

Heat is produced by the bird through normal metabolic activity, heat loss is achieved by evaporative loss during panting (birds do not have sweat glands). The effectiveness of the evaporative loss is diminished with a rise in relative humidity to the extent that at above 70%rh this ceases to function. It is worth remembering that the internal module temperature of a transportation module can be up to 10°C higher than the ambient environmental temperature.

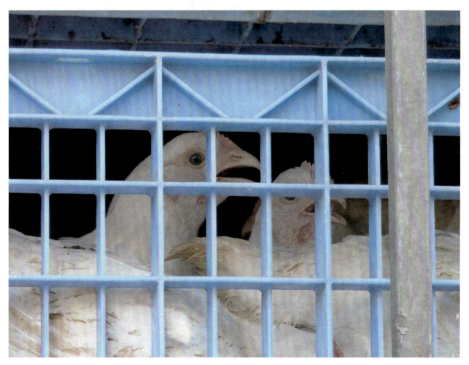

Panting birds in a transportation crate – evidence of thermal distress

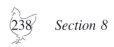

TRAUMA

N.B. Bruising is an indication of compromised welfare.

The title trauma indicates injury, be this bruising (haemorrhage), fractures of bones or dislocation of joints. It is important to understand that **trauma that occurs before the slaughter of the bird (ante mortem) will be associated with haemorrhage,** that which occurs after slaughter (post mortem) will not be associated with bleeding. The ability to recognise ante mortem trauma is of paramount importance, as this can be an indication that the welfare of the bird or flock has been compromised especially if the frequency of the lesions increases.

Bruising, or haemorrhage, occurs when blood vessels are ruptured and the contained blood leaks into surrounding tissue; this spread can be further exacerbated by the massage effect of the rubber plucking fingers. Damage to this vascular system can be caused by toxin and nutritional deficiency; however it is most commonly due to trauma. Any subcutaneous bruising can spread from the site of the initial injury as the skin in poultry is loosely connected to the underlying tissue. In the live animal, haemorrhage that is not fatal is eventually reabsorbed, resulting in a gradual change in colour of the bruising, a fact that can be used to approximate a timescale following the initial insult.

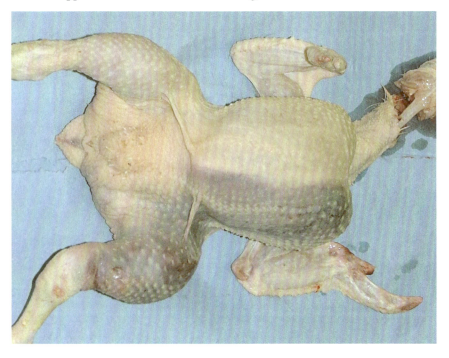

Haemorrhage due to fractured tibiotarsus. Note subcutaneous spread halted at skin attachment of sternum

Bruise colour	Approximate time since injury
Red	2 minutes
Red / purple	12 hours
Purple / green	24 hours
Green / Yellow	36 hours
Yellow	72 hours
Reabsorbing (no colour)	120 hours

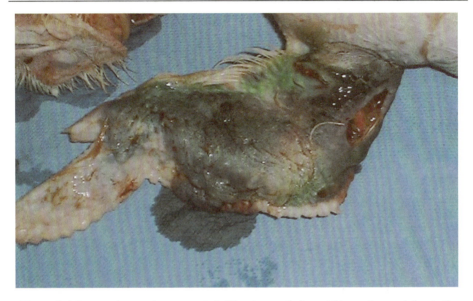

Traumatic injury to wing – colour suggests it did not occur during catching or transportation to the slaughterhouse

Extensive Bruising – Entire carcase unfit for human consumption.
Localised Bruising - Reject affected parts.
Superficial Bruising -   If less than 2cm in diameter and uncomplicated they may be left untrimmed.

FRACTURES

The avian skeleton has evolved to enable flight, extensive pneumatisation of the long bones by diverticula of the respiratory system is evident in all avian species. These adaptations are also present in broilers. Genetic selection has however produced broilers in which muscle growth exceeds bone formation to a degree that has produced an inherent weakness in the axial skeleton. The bones of the legs in particular, although retaining strength in the vertical plane, are prone to compound fracture when horizontal or rotational force is applied.

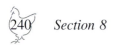

The most frequently observed point of fracture is the tibia, the femur possibly afforded greater protection by a larger surrounding muscle mass and proximity to the body. Fractures to the legs can occur due to the pivoting motion when placing birds into crates without support to the body during the catching operation, but other scenarios must be considered, such as sideways overextension by hangers struggling to keep up with line speed leading to greater force being applied to one leg.

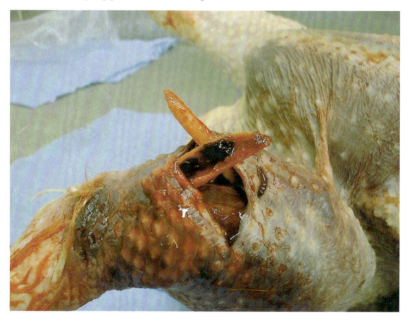

Compound fracture of the tibiotarsus

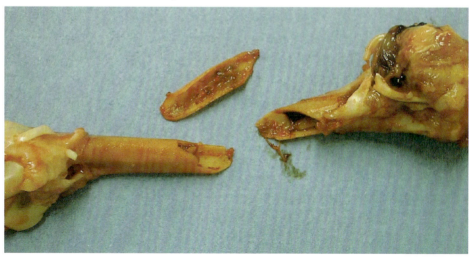

Dissected compound fracture of the tibiotarsus – illustrating thinness of compact bone layer

Fractures of the bones of the wing, particularly of the radius and ulna are found during post-mortem and ante mortem inspection. Wings can become trapped as drawers are shut during catching, and obstructed flapping by the bird can also lead to fracture of the bones if the object is struck by the wings in a right angled plane to the bones.

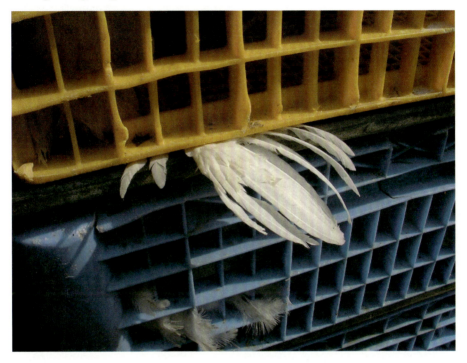

A wing trapped during the closing of a drawer

Fractures with haemorrhage – Affected tissues should be removed from the carcase at a joint, ensuring all affected tissue is removed.

Fractures without Haemorrhage breaking skin –Affected bone and muscle should be removed.

Fractures without haemorrhage not breaking skin –Straight break can be left. If bone fragments then trim as above.

DISLOCATION

The most frequently occurring dislocation found in broilers is the femur from the acetabulum of the pelvis and is often accompanied by massive haemorrhage due to the close association of the femoral artery. This dislocation can be partially linked to leg/joint weaknesses such as femoral head necrosis or femoral epiphysiolysis, but tends to be produced as a direct result of extreme abduction of the limb around this joint. This can occur with greater frequency in larger birds where the weight, possibly combined with single leg catching technique forces the femoral head from the acetabulum of the pelvis.

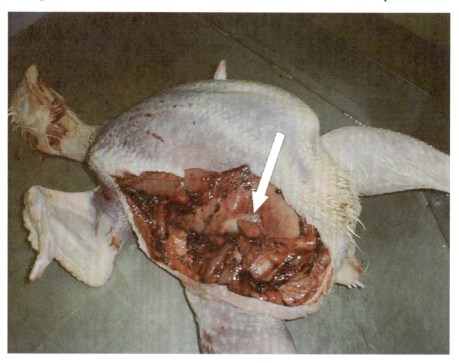

Dislocated femur (arrowed) note haemorrhaging that has become clotted

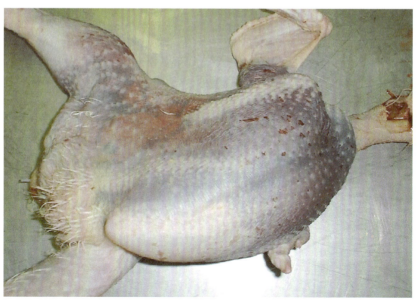

Massive haemorrhage associated with rupture of the femoral artery during dislocation

AUTOPSY
PROCEDURE

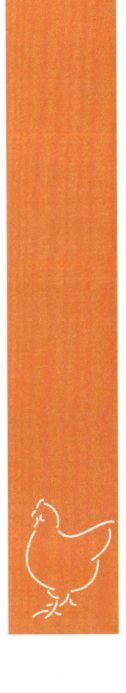

A post mortem examination (autopsy / necropsy), as opposed to a post mortem inspection (which basically endeavours to ascertain fitness for consumption), is a method of diagnosing a pathological condition from macroscopic lesions encountered. It is a procedure that is occasionally undertaken within the abattoir on birds discovered dead during ante mortem inspection, if only to ascertain whether the probability of death was due to disease or environmental/ processing conditions. Under these circumstances it is important to discover if any underlying pathological condition may have exacerbated the stress placed on the individual bird during catching, transportation and lairaging and therefore may have been a contributory factor in the death of the bird. This section describes a method for conducting a post mortem examination of a dead broiler; it is in no way intended to be definitive and is given as a guide. There are occasions when being able to conduct a post mortem examination on site is necessary and can be conducted with the minimum of equipment. It must be stressed that the post mortem only gives an indication of the cause of death or pathological condition and can normally only be confirmed by laboratory diagnosis which, if requested, will state the samples required and their condition.

The equipment used varies from person to person, scissors, a stout knife, bone shears, a bucket and a notepad and pen seem to suffice. The main piece of equipment required is knowledge; recognition of abnormality is provided by an appreciation of normality of organs and systems, an understanding of disease processes and how the bodily systems function and interrelate.

Once sample carcases have been selected (especially if feathered), place them, with the exception of the head, in a bucket of cold water containing detergent. The benefits of this are twofold. First, soaking the feathers prevents them from blowing around during examination; secondly the immersion cools the carcases slowing the rate of autolysis. If samples are to be sent whole for laboratory examination and diagnosis it is very important to cool them rapidly.

Remove upper beak by cutting through the nasal cavities. Check for signs of infection by squeezing this area and checking for the presence of fluid matter.

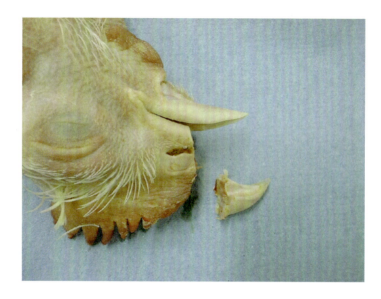

Cut through one corner of the mouth using scissors and cut down through the neck exposing the interior of the oesophagus.

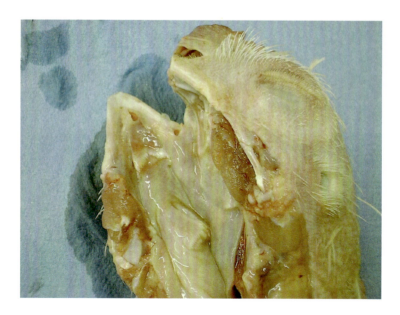

Examine the interior of the mouth for abnormalities.

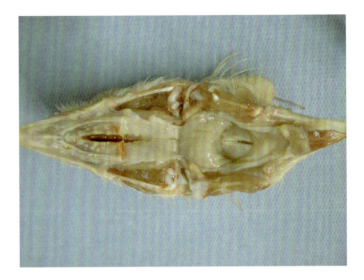

Make a shallow incision into the skin at the apex of the sternum. Extend the cut around the body on each side and then peel back the skin to expose the breast muscles.

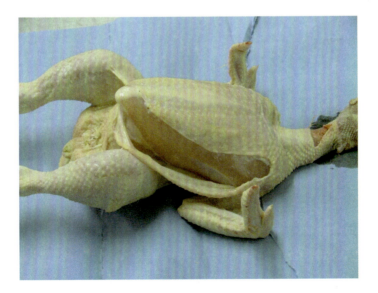

Examine the breast muscles, making note of their condition and colouring.

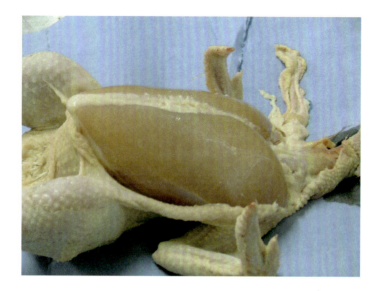

Cut the skin of the abdomen at the point of insertion of the legs. Press each leg down until the femur dislocates from the acetabulum and the legs lie flat.

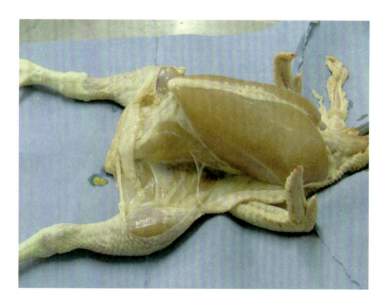

Remove the skin from the thighs and examine for petechial haemorrhages.

Examine the head of the femurs

Grasp the foot with the non-knife hand and making an oblique cut through the anterior third of the tibiotarsal bones, examine for tibial dyschondroplasia.

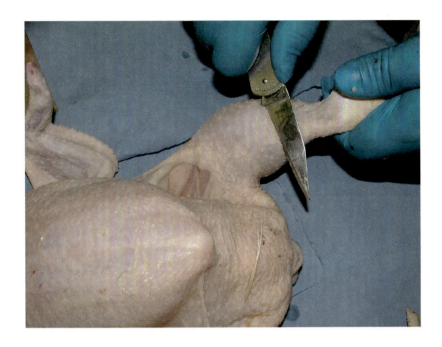

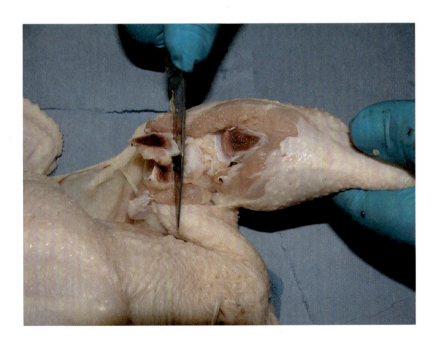

Make a shallow cut through the abdominal muscles at the apex of the sternum, ensure that the cut does not incise the abdominal organs within. Extend the cut through each of the pectoral muscles up to the shoulder joint each side.

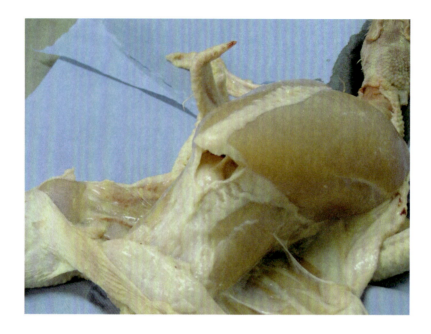

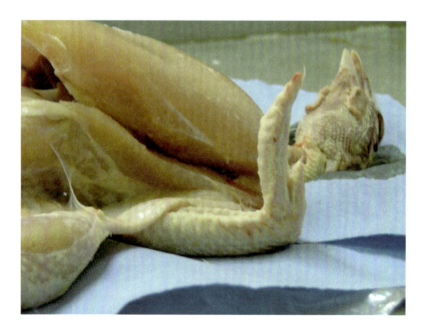

Using bone shears carefully cut through the ribs on either side, again ensuring that you do not damage the internal organs. Lift the sternum and dislocate the shoulder joints. Using the shears cut through the bones of the pectoral girdle and remove the sternum. Ensure that the crop (which adheres to the right hand side of the sternum) is not ruptured, by pulling it away from the breast with your fingers.

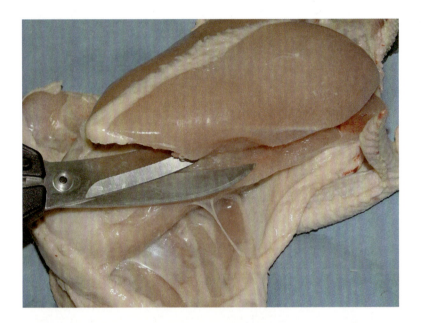

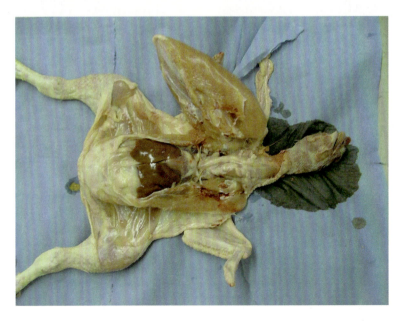

Examine the airsacs, liver and spleen for signs of abnormal colour, size, scarring and texture. Remove the liver carefully; remembering the gall bladder is attached to the duodenum by two ducts.

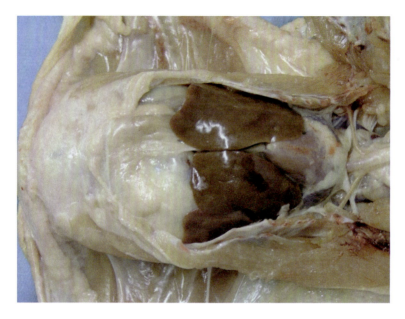

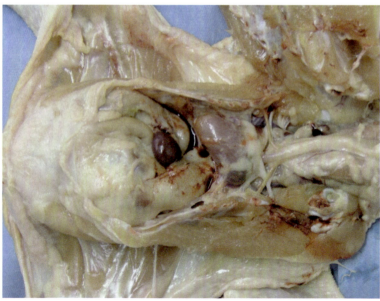

Check the pericardium and the heart. Remove the heart and the spleen.

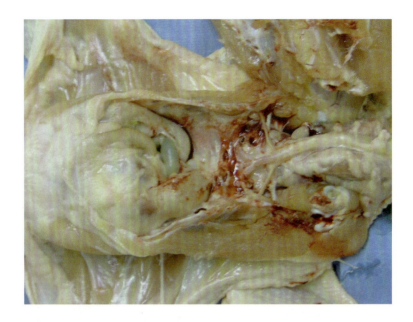

Cut the oesophagus at the neck and remove the digestive system by hand.

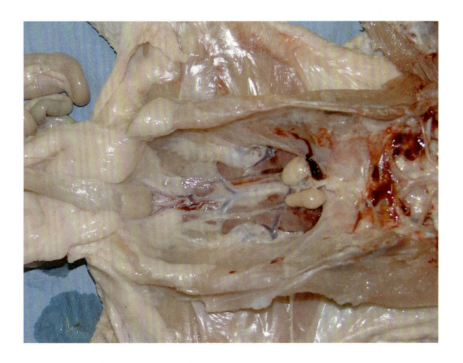

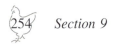

After checking the mesentery gently pull apart the digestive system.

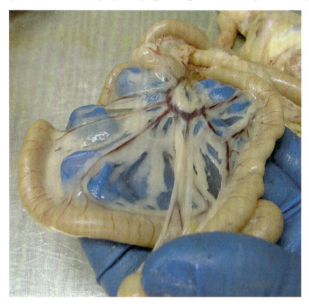

Using scissors cut the oesophagus down to the crop and examine the contents. Wash the crop and examine the lining.

Incise the proventriculus and gizzard. Remove contents and examine the lining of the proventriculus and the junction to the gizzard. Examine in detail the cutica gastrica of the gizzard for signs of erosion; check whether this lining can be peeled from the muscle. Examine the muscle.

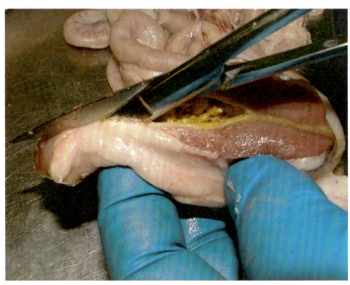

Examine the intestines for signs of haemorrhage and inflammation. If present note which third of the intestines is affected.

Examine the pancreas for signs of inflammation or atrophy.

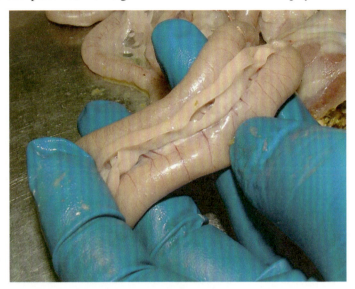

Open the duodenum and examine the contents noting any abnormalities. Wash out contents and examine the mucosal surface that should have a velvety texture.

Open the jejunum and ileum; examine the contents and the lining, paying particular attention to the area of the vitelline diverticulum.

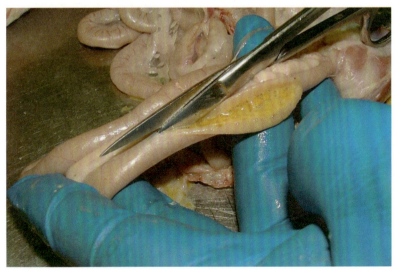

Observe the state of the caeca. Open the caeca paying particular attention to the state of the contents and their consistency. If haemorrhagic contents are found examine the lining of the caeca. Check the state of the caecal tonsils. Wash the contents on a piece of towel or in a plastic container, examine for the presence of worms.

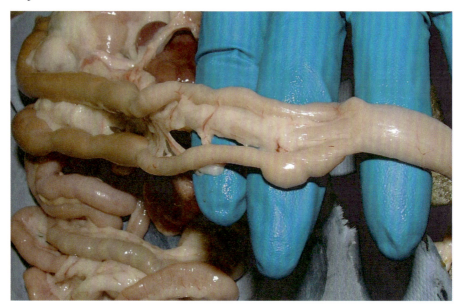

Open the colon and examine contents and lining.

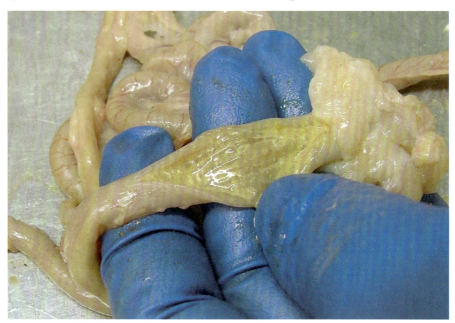

Examine the cloacal bursa, check for signs of enlargement or atrophy. Incise the bursa and examine lining for neoplastic growth and/or inflammation.

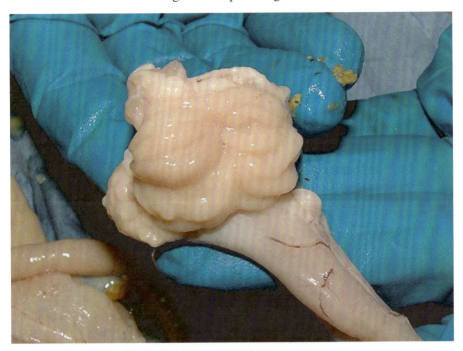

Using scissors open the trachea and examine the mucosa.

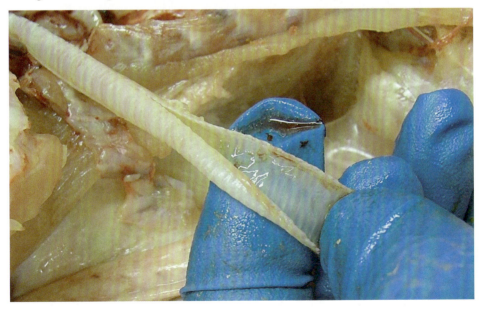

Examine the kidneys and ureters. Examine the testes and vas deferens, or the ovary and oviduct.

Using a blunt dissection technique, gently remove the kidneys to expose the lumbo-sacral plexus Compare each side for signs of inflammation.

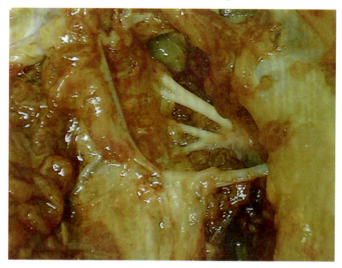

Remove the muscle group proximal to the femur of the thigh to expose the sciatic/ischiadic nerve that runs along the course of the femur. Check for signs of inflammation and remove the nerve. Under natural daylight check the nerve for loss of lateral striations.

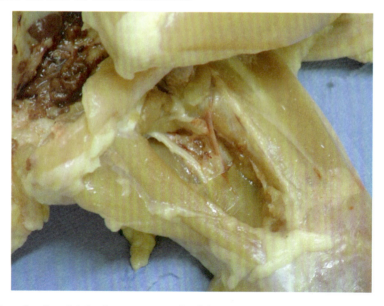

Examine the brachial plexus on each side, comparing the two nerve groups for signs of inflammation.

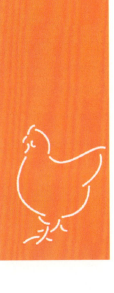

ANATOMY AIDE MEMOIRE

10

Axial Skeleton

Skull
Cervical
   vertebrae
Thoraic
   vertebrae
Pelvis
Synsacral
   vertebrae
Coccygeal
   vertebrae

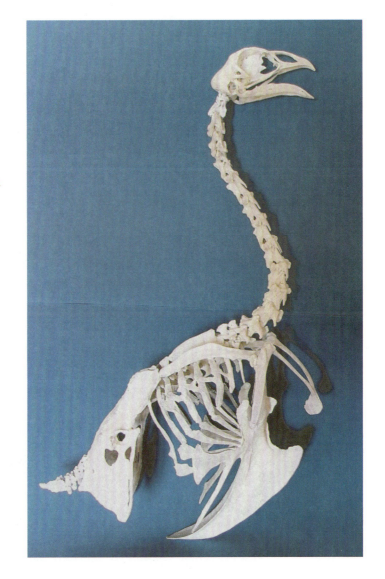

Pelvis

Pelvic bones ilium, ischium and pubis
Fused synsacral vertebrae

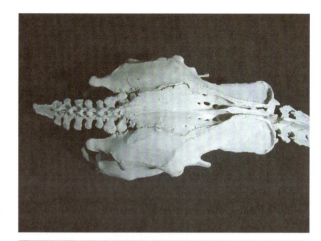

Sternum and Pectoral Girdle

2 clavicles producing furcula
2 scapula
2 coracoid

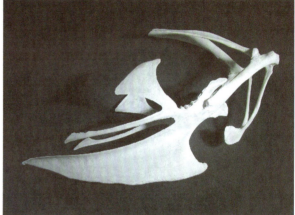

Wing
Humerus
Radius
Ulna
Radial carpal
Ulnal carpal
Metacarpals fused
3 digits

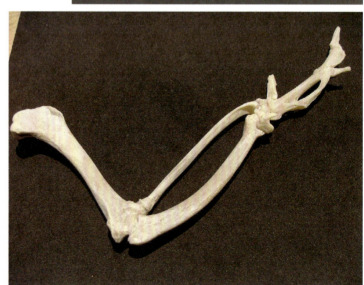

Leg

Femur
Patella
Tibiotarsus
Fibula
Metatarsus
Phlanges
  making up
  4digits

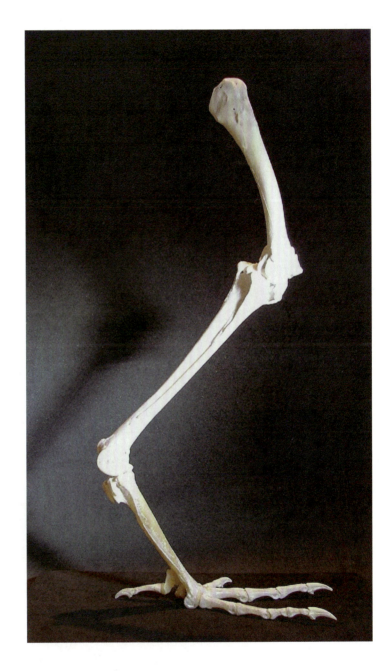

Lungs

Trachea
Syrinx
Bronchi
Lungs

Lungs non expansive.
Ridged on ventral surface
due to close association with
ribs

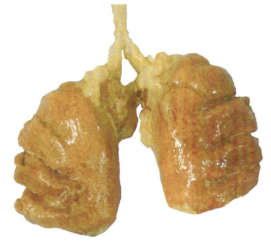

Airsacs

CHICKEN AIR SACS 9
Cervical 1 Pair, Interclavicular Fused, Anterior
Thoracic 1 pair, Posterior Thoracic 1 pair,
Abdominal 1 pair

TURKEY AIR SACS 7
Cervical Fused, Interclavicular 1 pair, Thoracic
1 pair, Abdominal 1 pair

DUCK AIR SACS 9
Cervical 1 pair, Interclavicular Fused, Anterior
Thoracic 1 pair, Posterior Thoracic 1 pair,
Abdominal 1 pair

Spleen

Chicken –
Spherical
Duck -
Pigeon -

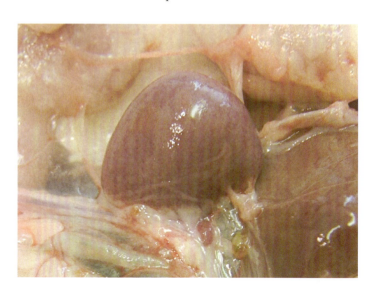

Heart

350-450
  beats per
  minute.
Normal fat
  deposit at
  apex.
Surrounded
  by
  pericardium

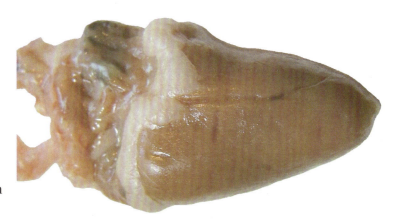

Liver

2 lobes
Gall bladder on
  visceral surface
  of right lobe
2 ducts take bile
  to the distal
  duodenum,
  hepatic duct
  and cystic duct

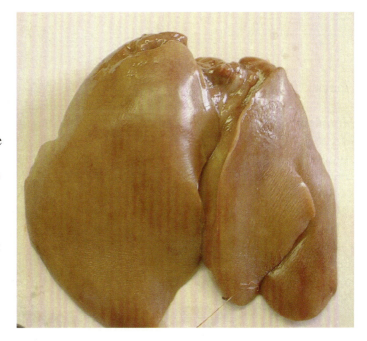

**Reproductive
System
Female**

Ovary
Infundibulum
Magnum
Isthmus
Uterus
Vagina
Cloaca

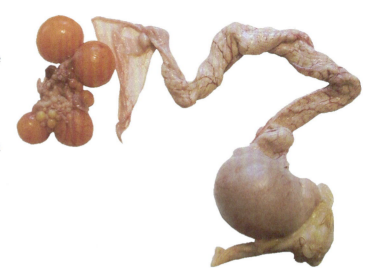

Cloaca

Cuprodeum
– faeces
Urodeum –
Urates
Proctodeum
– Gametes

B u r s a
opens into
proctodeum
and is site
of   B-cell
development

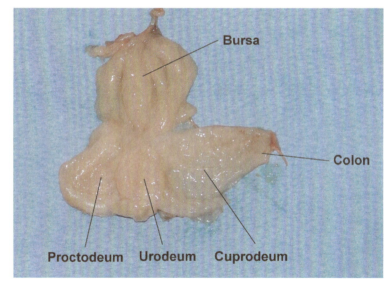

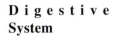

Digestive System

Mouth
Oesophagus
Crop
Oesophagus
Proventriculus
Gizzard
 (ventriculus)
Duodenum
Jejunum
Ileum
Caeca
Colon
Cloaca
Vent

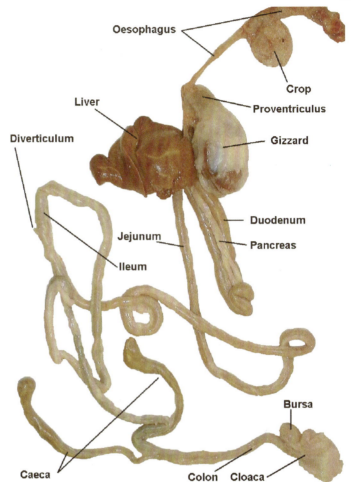

Oesophagus
Crop
Liver
Proventriculus
Diverticulum
Gizzard
Duodenum
Jejunum
Pancreas
Ileum
Bursa
Caeca
Colon
Cloaca

INDEX

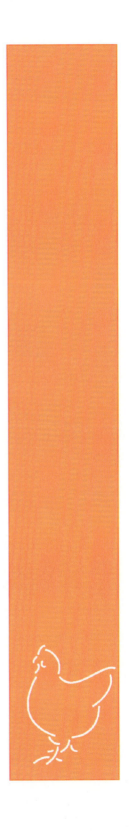

INDEX

A

A-band 20
Acetabulum 17
Acquired immune response 67
Actin 20
Adenosine triphosphate 20
Adenovirus 74
Adrenal gland 60
Adrenals 58
Affector cells 67
Aflatoxicosis. *See* Mycotoxicosis
Airsacculitis 163
Airsacs 36
Amyloidosis 76
Anasarca 168
Anatipestifer 76
Antibodies 67
Aortic rupture 76
Appendicular skeleton 16
Apteria 5
Arthritis 165
Ascaridia columbae 127
Ascaridia dissimilis 127
Ascaridia galli 127
Ascites 168
Aspergillosis 77
ATP. *See* Adenosine triphosphate
Atrium 41
Autotrophs 69
Avian chlamydiosis 78
Avian diphtheria. *See* Fowl pox
Avian influenza 78
Avian keratoacanthoma 141
Avian leukosis 138
Avian malignant oedema. *See* Gangrenous dermatitis

Avian mMycoplasmosis 79. *See also* Infectious synovitis
Avian pneumoencephalitis. *See* Newcastle disease
Avian rhinotracheitis. *See* Swollen head syndrome
Avian salmonellosis 79
Avian tuberculosis 80
Axial skeleton 8
Axon 55

B

B-cells 67
Benign tumours 135
Big liver disease. *See* Avian leukosis
Bile staining 231
Binary fission 69
Biotin deficiency 180
Birnavirus 74
Blood vessels 42, 43
Bluecomb. *See* Transmissible enteritis of turkeys
Body lice 129
Botulism 80
Brachial cysts 226
Brain 55
Breast blister 81
Breast blisters 208
Breast burn 212
Bronchi 23
Brooder pneumonia. *See* Aspergillosis
Bruising 238
Bumblefoot 176
Burrowing flea. *See* *Echidnophaga gallinacea*
Bursa of Fabricius 51